After Brain Injury
Telling Your Story

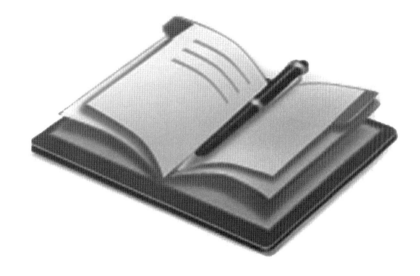

A Journaling Workbook

Barbara Stahura
Susan B. Schuster, M.A., CCC-SLP

Library of Congress Control Number: 2009935810

Copyright © 2009 Lash & Associates Publishing/Training Inc.

Lash & Associates Publishing/Training Inc. gives permission to the purchaser to copy activity worksheets. Copies may not be sold or published in any other form.

Published by Lash & Associates Publishing/Training Inc.
708 Young Forest Drive, Wake Forest, NC 27587
Tel: & Fax: (919) 562-0015

This book is part of a series on brain injury among children, veterans and adults. For a free catalog, contact Lash & Associates
Tel. & Fax (919) 562-0015 or visit our web site www.lapublishing.com

ISBN 9781931117524

$30.00 US

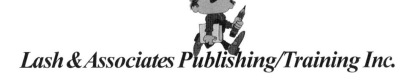

Advance Praise for
After Brain Injury: Telling Your Story

"*After Brain Injury: Telling Your Story* by Barbara Stahura and Susan B. Schuster is a landmark book for people with brain injury and their friends and family. The authors provide a compelling roadmap to help guide survivors to understand the ways that brain injury can affect their lives. This is a beautifully written and thoughtful book that should be embraced by anyone who deals with the aftermath of brain injury." – James W. Pennebaker, Professor of Psychology, University of Texas at Austin

"Through this book, people learn tools for self-discovery, healing and moving forward. The exercises demonstrate enormous empathy for and understanding of the individual with a brain injury and with that, hopefulness and a sense of worth. This is a very welcome contribution to the brain injury self-help literature and one that I will share with my son who is 13 years post injury." – Linda Robinson, Trauma Research Manager, Inova Regional Trauma Center, Falls Church, VA and former Director of Education and Research at the Brain Injury Association of America, Alexandria, VA

"This is a wonderful and important book. It covers the whole gamut of starting one's life over after a TBI and how to approach all aspects of that readjustment. It is so timely, especially with the men and women I am dealing with out of our two current wars." – Floyd "Shad" Meshad, founder and president, National Veterans Foundation

"With remarkable clarity and grace, the authors bring the healing power of journal writing to the experience of brain injury. Every page brims with compassionate guidance through well-designed writing processes, real-life examples, and a running voice of encouragement. A welcome addition to the body of literature in journal therapy." – Kathleen Adams LPC, Director, Center for Journal Therapy and Author, *Journal to the Self*

"Stahura and Schuster make the path so much easier with a practical introspective vision that uses the creative power of the journal. This book should be very widely used by those with brain injuries. These authors definitely have a healing presence." – Stephen G. Post, Director, Center for Medical Humanities, Compassionate Care and Bioethics, Stony Brook University

"*After Brain Injury: Telling Your Story* provides a practical guide of ideas and suggestions for transitioning through the life-changing events of surviving a traumatic brain injury (TBI). With the increasing incidence of traumatic brain injury in the general and military populations, this book is a useful tool for both therapists and family members." – Sandra L. Schneider, Ph.D. BC-NCD, Department of Hearing and Speech Sciences at Vanderbilt University School of Medicine and Director of the Pi Beta Phi Rehabilitation Institute

"This book will provide a great tool and guide to all people who help those with brain injuries, whether that be family members or professionals. As brother of someone with a brain injury, it helps me understand more of what she goes through and what could help her to not lose sight of all the gifts she has to offer, including the richness of her life story. I intend to share this book with her!" – John Fox, CPT, *Poetic Medicine: The Healing Art of Poem-making*

"Stahura and Schuster have a detailed understanding of the many issues that arise during the struggle to reconstruct lives disrupted by brain injury. They couple that understanding with their experience helping survivors to use journaling as a tool to gain insight, comfort, and direction. The authors offer overviews of the issues and provide related prompts for journaling, first done with guidance in a workshop setting, but clearly able to be self-directed as part of a survivor's regular life practice." – Lynne Oland, MSN, PhD Research Scientist, Dept. of Neuroscience, University of Arizona, Tucson, AZ

Disclaimer

A great deal of care has been taken to provide accurate and current information in this book. However, every brain injury is as individual as the person who experiences it. Therefore, the ideas, suggestions, general principles, and conclusions presented in this book are subject to your personal health and sound medical advice. We cannot present every possibility, nor do we presume that any or all possibilities in this book relate to your situation.

This book is sold with the understanding that neither the authors nor the publisher are engaged in rendering psychological, financial, legal, or other professional services. If medical assistance or expert counseling is needed, please seek the services of a competent professional.

Table of Contents

Dedication..vii
Acknowledgements..viii
Foreward..ix
Introduction..1
The Importance of Story...3
What is Journaling?..6

Chapter 1 After Brain Injury: What Happened? What Can I Discover?.................13
1-1	How My Injury Happened..14
1-2	How It Feels to be Me..15
1-3	The Worst Part...16
1-4	Making Metaphor..17
1-5	Talking with Your Brain..18
1-6	Map to My True Self...20
1-7	Kindred Spirits, or Not..21
1-8	What Else Happened to Me?..22

Chapter 2 Loss and Change: Brain Power, Memory, and More................................23
- 2-1 Loss List..24
- 2-2 Empty Spaces...25
- 2-3 Unnamed Losses..26
- 2-4 Glued Together...27
- 2-5 Off Balance...28
- 2-6 Memory...29
- 2-7 Memory Lists..31
- 2-8 Improving Memory..32
- 2-9 Other Functions Lost..33
- 2-10 Because of These Losses..34
- 2-11 Resilience...35
- 2-12 I Still Have This...37
- 2-13 Using the Senses to Remember..38

Chapter 3 Relationships: Family, Friends, and Others..41
- 3-1 Once Upon a Time...42
- 3-2 Explaining My Injury...43
- 3-3 Understanding..44
- 3-4 Writing a Letter...45
- 3-5 What I Really Need..47
- 3-6 Confusing Changes..48
- 3-7 Loneliness...49
- 3-8 Overcoming Loneliness..50
- 3-9 Asking for Help, Part 1...51
- 3-10 Asking for Help, Part 2...53

Chapter 4 Adjustments: Anger and Grief..55
- 4-1 Telling the Story of My Anger..56
- 4-2 Feeling the Anger...57
- 4-3 Grieving the Losses...59

4-4	Feeling the Grief	61
4-5	Comfort	62
4-6	Awareness, Acceptance, Acknowledgement, and Accommodation	63

Chapter 5 Back Into the Community: Moving Forward With Hope 67

5-1	What Your Life Means	68
5-2	Hope in Your Future	69
5-3	Nurturing Hope	71
5-4	Asking Others to Hope With You	72
5-5	Your Home	73
5-6	A Letter from Home	74
5-7	New People	75
5-8	Making Your Way Around	77
5-9	Work Issues	78
5-10	Back at Work	80
5-11	Back to School	81
5-12	Social Activities	82
5-13	Giving of Yourself	83

Chapter 6 Later On: Any Positives? 85

6-1	Your "Sports Pages"	87
6-2	Your Better Stories	88
6-3	Time Capsule Treasures, Part 1	90
6-4	Time Capsule Treasures, Part 2	91
6-5	No One Can Take This Away From Me	92
6-6	Invitation	93
6-7	RSVP	94
6-8	Learning From Your "Teachers"	95
6-9	Being a Teacher	97

Chapter 7 Miscellaneous Prompts 99

Chapter 8 Journaling in a Group 103

Brain Injury Resources 105

Sample Journaling Pages 107

Dedication

To Ken, who continues to love and teach me so much as we travel together through life and the mysteries of brain injury. – Barbara Stahura

In memory of my father, Bernard L. Schuster (4-26-26 to 12-24-08), my biggest inspiration and survivor of a cerebral aneurysm, who taught me through words—and most importantly, by example—that service to others is one's greatest aspiration and purpose. – Susan B. Schuster

Acknowledgements

We offer our heartfelt thanks to Mindy Tharan, who suggested in 2006 that we create a writing workshop for people with brain injury. She planted the seed that first grew to assist a small group of people with brain injuries in Tucson and is now bearing fruit for many others we will never meet.

Martha Gerganoff, CEO of HealthSouth Rehabilitation Hospital of Southern Arizona, also played an essential role in the creation of this book. When we asked her if we could hold our first journaling workshop at her facility, just to see if it would work, she opened her arms in welcome. It worked, and as of this writing, she welcomes us still. Thank you, Martha.

Our workshop, also titled "After Brain Injury: Telling Your Story," has been attended by enthusiastic participants, each willing to journal from their hearts in order to learn more about themselves and their brain injuries, and to help themselves—and one another—recover further. We thank them for their courage, curiosity, and honesty, as well as for their journal entries included in this book.

We thank Steven Gurgevich, Ph.D., for his kind and wise advice regarding the structure of parts of this book. Barbara also thanks him for the guidance he has offered in the wake of Ken's brain injury.

Thanks also to the many survivors over the years who have let us be part of their recovery journey. We have learned so much from them, and their inspiration is reflected in this book.

Thank you to our many teachers and mentors who have provided wisdom and background for our personal growth in doing this project.

Thanks to Joyce Thomas for her patient and thorough proofreading.

Susan would also like to give personal appreciation to two individuals: Her mother, DaLene Schuster, who gave her so much encouragement and input in her younger writing endeavors, and to Barbara Stahura, without whom this book would not have come to be.

Foreword

By John W. Richards, MSW, MBA, LICSW & TBI survivor

How do people come back after sustaining a traumatic brain injury? What are the ingredients and activities that we can pursue as we try to put ourselves and our lives back together? What are the methods and strategies to help us think about, reflect on, examine and consider our feelings, thoughts and dreams? How can we meet the challenges and grow as we try to reassemble ourselves and create a new life post-injury?

As anyone who has walked the path of recovery of traumatic or acquired brain injury (TBI or ABI), or who has supported others to walk along the journey of recovery knows, recovery just isn't easy. It doesn't matter how severe or "mild"[1] the injury may be. The best metaphor I have ever come across for my own TBI recovery was that it was about as easy as climbing Mt. Everest....if I started in New Hampshire!

Most people in the United States today have little to no awareness of the "silent epidemic" of brain injuries. **Traumatic brain injury is the leading cause of death and disability among children and young adults.**

Nor is brain injury on the mind at all of the 1.3 million [2] people who will sustain a brain injury this year in the United States. Nor is it on the mind of their families or friends who will at some time spend countless hours in waiting rooms, in intensive care units and emergency departments wondering what to do next and how to proceed from here. What does it all mean? How and how well will their loved one recover?

In this thoughtful and reflective discussion of journaling after a brain injury, Barbara Stahura and Susan B. Schuster offer a strong and worthy guide that can effectively help in the journey of recovery. The authors have tackled a difficult and complex subject effectively and with compassion. Most importantly, they thoroughly and thoughtfully approach the question of, "What factors create and contribute to an optimal recovery?" They focus on encouraging survivors to do their best to think about and reflect on their specific responses through journaling.

Having worked as a clinical social worker and human service administrator for many years, I was shocked one day when I woke up (literally) in a Vail bed in a brain injury trauma hospital. I heard that I had experienced a "brain bleed" and had a long recovery to face, although that information made no sense to me at the time. I intellectually understood the term "recovery" from my family and caregivers' words. But I certainly did NOT truly emotionally understand that I had had a traumatic brain injury, nor how my life would change in the coming years.

Here I was the capable, healthy, energetic president of a human service agency and president of the board of directors of the Brain Injury Association of New Hampshire. HOW could this have happened, **to me**? Further, I did not begin to truly understand the reality of the challenges facing me over the coming years for a LOOONNNGGGG time.

Most people in the United States today have little or no awareness of the "silent epidemic" of brain injuries, nor of the challenging realities of their new life. There are 3.1 million people in the United States alone[3] who live with both visible and "invisible" disabilities that began with a brain injury. In fact, a common saying in the "brain injury community" is...

"Brain injury isn't anything at all,
never even anything on your mind,
until it's the only thing on your mind."

I was quite fortunate, indeed, in the resources for my recovery that were provided to me — medically, socially, and for rehabilitation. But I still found the early stages of recovery overwhelming and confusing on a daily basis. In retrospect, if I had utilized the strategy of journaling during the earlier stages of recovery, that tool may have greatly assisted my short term memory deficit, a common challenge for many survivors. Journaling would also have been valuable in improving organizational systems and my emotional outlook and awareness. I personally believe that anyone who retains a level of awareness after such an injury is certain to face some level of depression when thinking about what they have lost.

Ms. Stahura and Ms. Schuster obviously know of what they speak and have done a thorough, detailed and organized overview of many of the countless issues that arise during recovery from brain injury.

One of the many strengths of journaling is that it represents an effective means for a survivor to review and track progress over time. In the long slow doldrums of the recovery journey, looking back at one's journal can be a highly effective means of assessing and staying aware of one's progress. Of uppermost importance in the recovery journey is the challenge of generating and fostering **resiliency** – one of the overall most essential components of re-creation, and on which the authors focus particular attention.

If you have never sustained a brain injury, or if no one in your family has, do everything in your power to keep it that way! Prevention is key. If you or your loved one is a survivor, think about bringing journaling into your life as you slowly walk the long road of recovery.

[1] An odd and misleading bit of nomenclature.
[2] Centers for Disease Control
[3] Estimate from the Centers for Disease Control

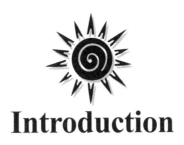

Introduction

*"'What is your medicine?' I was asked.
'Story. Story is my medicine,' I answered."*
Deena Metzger, Entering the Ghost River

Telling Your Story

As a person with a brain injury, you have been hurt and traumatized by something most people haven't experienced and can't understand. Whether your brain injury is the result of an accident, surgery, military service, violence, infection, medical emergency, or any other cause, you now must deal with a number of challenges you never expected or imagined. One major challenge you face is making sense of a life disrupted and perhaps altered forever. Another is being accepted as a person who still has value and whose life still holds meaning and purpose. Yet another is revealing a new self to people, perhaps even your loved ones, who don't realize or understand the changes the injury caused in you (changes you may not understand, either). Since every brain injury is as unique as the person who experienced it, you will face your own individual hurdles.

However, no matter how many challenges your brain injury has created for you, one thing is certain: You have a new story to tell.

Being natural-born storytellers, we humans assign meaning to everything. So, usually without realizing it, we build our lives from the stories we tell ourselves and each other. Like weavers, we combine ordinary and significant events alike into stories that tell us who we are and where we belong in our world. When we answer the question, "What did you do at work/school/home today?" we are telling our story. When we describe our honeymoon in Hawaii or how we watched the polar bears at the nearby zoo, that's a story. So is writing a letter that reveals our sorrow over the death of a baby son or the quiet joy of a long-lasting love. When we dream of a desired future or struggle to understand our past, we are using storytelling to shape our lives. We also hold many unspoken stories in the deepest chambers of our hearts and spirits, some of which can embrace us like a lullaby or burn us like acid.

Creating a New Story

An injury to the magnificent, mysterious brain can upset the familiar story of a life in ways no other injury or illness can. You may face not only challenges with your physical abilities but, more essentially, you may find yourself wrestling with difficult mental and emotional changes. So much you knew about yourself—the wealth of information you depended upon to lead your life—can blur or disappear, leaving you stranded and struggling in an unknown place. You can feel as though you've been kidnapped to an alien planet where nothing is familiar, where you feel threatened and lost. You might even feel as though you have disappeared.

Fortunately, story can be your medicine, as Deena Metzger says. Creating a new story after your injury can allow a measure of healing (even years later), help rebuild your life, and offer much-needed hope. Like laying stones to form a path, you can use your own words and insights to guide you through a now unfamiliar world. By giving voice to your deepest self after the trauma of a brain injury, to whatever extent you are able, you can forge a new understanding.

Journaling to Tell Your Story

One powerful method of telling your own story is a simple writing technique called journaling. It allows you to express your innermost thoughts on the page, free of judgment from anyone else—and without any requirement to correct and revise your writing (journaling is *not* a test!). You can journal in only minutes a day, several times a week or a month, or you can spend more time. You can keep your writing private or later share it with others. You can write while you're alone or as part of a group.

In a journaling group, participants often choose to read their entries aloud. In the small journaling groups the authors have led, we have found that this kind of sharing opens the door to companionship among the participants, whose brain injuries have often left them feeling isolated. They have told us how much more connected and valuable they feel after sharing their journal entries, since other people with brain injury can identify with the obstacles, challenges, and hard-won successes they write about. In addition, since the participants have reached various levels of recovery, the support also encourages the more recently injured members to keep up the good fight for recovering as much as they can.

However, whether you write on your own or in a group, and whether you share your journal entries or keep them private, the important thing is that you give *yourself* permission to write them. Without that, your story will remain undiscovered.

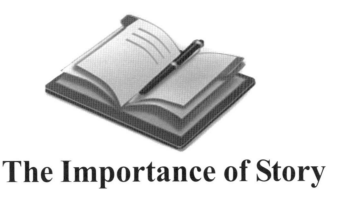

The Importance of Story

*"Humans are not ideally set up to understand logic;
they are ideally set up to understand stories."*
Roger C. Shank, cognitive scientist

*"We make our lives bigger or smaller, more expansive or more limited,
according to the interpretation of life that is our story."*
Christina Baldwin
*Storycatcher: Making Sense of Our Lives Through
the Power and Practice of Story*

What is a Story?

This book is titled *After Brain Injury: Telling Your Story*. What is story? Why is it important?

Often, "story" means pieces of writing such as science fiction or fairy tales or romance novels. But in this book, it means the story of your life, all those millions of pieces, large and small, that have gathered together to become "You." That huge, complex story begins with the basic facts of your life: for instance, where and when you were born, your gender and ethnicity, the age of your parents and their marital status at that time, whether they died young or lived into old age, the number and ages of your siblings, whether you have a religious faith, where and when you attended school, and illnesses and injuries.

On the day you were born, you began the lifelong process of collecting and creating stories about yourself and the world. Especially in the youngest years, this is mostly an unconscious process, since your young brain basically soaks up whatever happens to and around you.

Stories of Your Life

Later, you understand yourself through the filter of what you unknowingly absorbed. Far more important than the "facts" or outward events and experiences of your life are the ways your mind, heart, and spirit interpret them. *Your interpretations are the stories you live by*.

For example, when parents divorce, young children often believe they are the cause of the split. They experience the painful fact that their parents no longer live together, and because they don't yet understand the world of adults, they can automatically interpret the divorce as their fault. Obviously, this can create psychological and emotional havoc for them, which has the potential to affect the rest of their lives. Fortunately, caring parents can transform that interpretation by gently explaining that the children are in no way responsible.

This automatic interpreting of events does not disappear when we grow up. Say you're driving in rush hour traffic, already feeling stressed, when a car barrels out of a parking lot directly in front of you. You jam on your brakes with inches to spare. Startled and angry, you yell (or worse) at the other driver because you interpreted his act as stupidity combined with poor driving skills. You carry your anger home, where you yell at your children for no reason they can see, which upsets them. However, what if the other driver had just received word that his daughter had been severely injured and was rushing to the hospital when he left the parking lot? That does not excuse his actions behind the wheel, but they become more understandable. If you had known that fact, you might have interpreted his actions differently and felt compassion for him.

Remember also that when people's personal stories combine and interact, they form the field that grows the world's stories, which can span many centuries. Just as trillions of cells gather together to create one body, many tiny stories give rise to an enormous one. And just as an individual's story interpretations are crucial, the same is true for the world.

Imagine a grocery bag full of food. A person—or a culture—could mindlessly fill it with junk food that does nothing to nourish and may even do harm. Alternatively, the bag could be packed with nutritious, delicious foods that support health and vitality for many decades. The stories you believe—about anything—are your emotional food. If you repeatedly berate yourself with negative labels, you live one story. If you instead often remind yourself that you're smart and worthy, that you're fine just the way you are, you live another. If you hold a belief that prevents you from attempting a new activity, you live a different story than if you tried and succeeded, or if you tried and failed and tried again. All of these beliefs create various stories that can take your life in many directions.

The Story of Brain Injury

So it is with the story of brain injury itself. The old "official" story said that any possible recovery would occur in the first six months, or one year, or two years tops. After that time period, further recovery was believed nearly impossible. In this version, people who may have made great strides with further rehabilitation and therapy were often cut off, leaving them unable to fulfill the potential they might otherwise have had.

Fortunately, science has transformed that old story. Brain researchers recently have discovered that the human brain is far more capable of recovery, and for many additional years, than was previously believed. This does not mean everyone with a brain injury will recover or continue to make progress—that depends on the actual injury and a variety of other factors—but it does offer hope of further healing and restoration of function, with improved possibilities for a better post-injury life.

Sharing Your Story

Telling your stories is a way to exchange knowledge and insights and to build a sense of community. It helps you learn to cope with new situations and to make decisions. It is also vital. You need to be able to express yourself in open and honest ways for your mental, emotional, spiritual, and even physical health. Yes, it can be devastating when a person important to you ignores the story you're trying to tell, but when someone *really* listens with care and understanding, the magic of being heard can make you bloom. Sharing your stories with compassionate listeners strengthens and validates you—even if you are the only listener. Telling your stories can heal you, and it can heal those who hear them.

After a terrible trauma such as a brain injury, telling your stories about that experience can help you release bottled-up emotions that may be confusing or harmful. Telling your stories can lead you to an understanding of what has happened to you, why you feel so different, and why parts of your life are so changed. It also can foster understanding in your family and friends, employers and co-workers, as well as many others, because they have been affected, too—your story has influenced the world's.

A brain injury can turn a life upside down. Before it, you had one story of your life. After it, you began a new and unfamiliar one. How do you learn to live within this new reality? If you can't go back to the way you were, how do you figure out who you can be now? The answer: you tell your story, and it will show you how.

The Story of Your Life

By creating new stories of your life, you can reconstruct or re-energize it. You give yourself the opportunity to improve in those areas that no longer work well, and also build upon the strengths you have. You can use what you *do* know to create something you don't yet know.

Here's another quote from Christina Baldwin, "Something is happening in the power and practice of story: In the midst of overwhelming noise and distraction, the voice of story is calling us to remember our true selves."

With *After Brain Injury: Telling Your Story*, you can bring clarity to some of your old stories and also create new ones. You can begin to uncover and sort out issues related to your brain injury that affect the current Story of Your Life. By using this workbook you can begin to remember your true self, that essential part of you that never changes, even after the "overwhelming noise and distraction" of a brain injury. You can do this by learning how to journal.

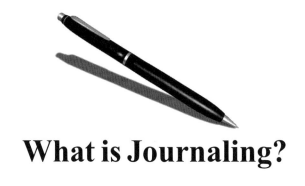

What is Journaling?

"...writing can make pain tolerable, confusion clearer and the self stronger."
Anna Quindlen, *Newsweek*, Jan. 22, 2007

To journal is to write about your life—it is telling your story. Furthermore, "life-based writing is one of the most reliable and effective ways to heal, change and grow," according to Kathleen Adams, author of *Journal to the Self* and founder/director of The Center for Journal Therapy.

Listening to Yourself

You constantly "talk" to yourself with your thoughts, but when you take a few moments to journal, you're also listening. As you write, you retrieve information from the rich storehouse of your subconscious mind and imagination. Once recorded on the page, your words become useful in the continuing creation of your new, post-injury story.

With journaling, you can explore all aspects of your life and the emotions connected to them. You can grieve or shout with joy. You can let your writing take you wherever your mind, heart, spirit, and imagination want to go. You can expand your creativity, help yourself heal, and build self-confidence. You can uncover memories that may help you understand the chaos of the present. You can vent. You can break loose from old obstacles and traumas that are holding you back. You can begin to create your future by imagining yourself there. You can follow a path that leads you inward to heart-places where you have never before traveled. With patience and time, your journal writing will empower you as it transports you to deeper levels of self-understanding.

Writing and Healing

The healing, change, and growth that come from journaling can appear on the physical, emotional, mental, and spiritual levels. (Remember that these "parts" of us cannot be separated, so whatever affects one affects them all.) Psychologist James Pennebaker has long researched the links between expressing emotions through writing and healing, and his work provides some surprising information about the mind-body connection. He has conducted many studies in which people wrote about traumatic or stressful events for twenty minutes daily over several days. In this free-flowing writing, people kept their pens moving steadily and didn't worry about grammar or punctuation. Based on blood tests administered before and after the days of writing, Dr. Pennebaker and his colleagues found that participants had stronger immune systems for up to several weeks afterward. The writers also scored higher in psychological well-being, functioned better in daily tasks, took fewer medications, and had lower pain levels.

Another journaling study was reported in the *Journal of the American Medical Association* (April 14, 1999). People with rheumatoid arthritis or asthma wrote for twenty minutes daily for three days in a row about traumas in their past. Four months later, nearly half showed significant improvement in their illnesses. In the control group, which wrote about more mundane topics, only a quarter of the people showed similar progress.

In another study, people who had cancer did "expressive writing exercises"—similar to journaling—for 20 minutes over several days about how their illness had changed them and how they felt about it. They reported that the writing helped to ease their stress about the cancer.

Journaling also has been shown to improve mental health in people with panic attacks and eating disorders, or who were victims of sexual abuse.

Why does journaling about traumatic events have a positive effect on physical ailments? Dr. Pennebaker believes that "actively holding back or inhibiting our thoughts and feelings can be hard work. Over time, the work of inhibition gradually undermines the body's defenses." On the other hand, "…writing or talking about upsetting things can influence our basic values, our daily thinking patterns, and feelings about ourselves. In short, there appears to be something akin to an urge to confess. Not disclosing our thoughts and feelings can be unhealthy. Divulging them can be healthy." (*Opening Up: The Healing Power of Expressing Emotions*, James W. Pennebaker, Ph.D., The Guilford Press, 1990 and 1997)

Fortunately, this healthy divulging can be accomplished on paper, and it does not require involving another person—the only confidante you need is your journal.

But don't think that your journal is a place for writing only about difficult or traumatic circumstances. In fact, it's been found that people who journal over long periods only about the bad times end up feeling worse rather than better. So be sure to record positive, happy events and situations as well. Just as your life has many facets, so should your journal.

Even though the authors of this book know of no studies yet reported with people with brain injury who journal, many other studies make clear that anyone can benefit from the practice. Throughout this book, you will see examples of journal entries. Most of them were written by people with brain injury, some of whom requested that we not use their real names. In the spontaneous spirit of journal writing, we left their original thoughts intact, including "creative" spelling and sometimes mismatched words. (If clarification was necessary, those words appear in brackets: [xxx].) A few entries were composed by the authors based on their experiences living with a person with a brain injury, leading journaling workshops, and providing speech and cognitive therapy for many years. All the journal entries appear in `Courier font`.

Journaling Tips

There is no right or wrong way to journal. You can adapt the process to suit yourself and your abilities. However, here are some tips that can help you get the most out of it.

For your eyes only

What you write in your journal is meant for no one's eyes but yours. As you write, don't fret about anyone judging your words, or you. Just go for it!

Write without rules

This writing is not graded and it's not meant for publication, so don't worry about spelling, punctuation, or grammar. If you spend time deciding where to put a comma or puzzling over spelling, that kind of intellectual processing stops the spirit-centered flow and can dam up the magic and mystery trying to emerge. As much as possible, let your hand write whatever it wants to write.

Write often

If you can, write in your journal frequently. If you write daily or several times a week, you will find it easier to stay in the journaling flow over time. You may grow so fond of it, you may come to miss it if you skip a day! However, only you can determine your best writing schedule, so write when you are moved to write.

Write by hand

If at all possible, use a pen or pencil to write your journaling entries. For some reason, the physical act of writing seems to open up the mind and allow more access to creativity and insights. However, if your brain injury or another disability prevents you from using a writing instrument, or if you prefer to use a computer, do so. If you are not able to type, you can speak your responses into a recording device (many inexpensive recorders are available) or use voice-recognition software on your computer. You can also ask a trusted person—friend, family member, or counselor, for instance—to write your responses as you speak them. (Thank you to John Fox, CPT, for this suggestion.) A few of the exercises in this book require crayons or colored markers, but if you're not able to draw, you can still respond to the prompts that accompany the drawing.

Try freewriting

Use the technique called freewriting if possible. This means you put your pen on the paper and keep going. Aim for 10 to 20 minutes, and set a timer or alarm if you have one. However, just a few minutes will work if you're pressed for time or that's what your abilities allow. If at all possible, keep your hand on the page, and keep it moving for the whole time. If you come to a dead end for a moment, you can write something like, "I'm stuck, I'm stuck," or repeat your last few words. New thoughts will appear soon for you to write. Freewriting lets insights come to light that otherwise might never appear in your conscious mind, and they are like gold nuggets—something valuable worth waiting for.

Go with the flow

Don't plan ahead what you'll write, and don't force yourself to be logical. Just write whatever rises up. When you get into the flow of the writing, it's almost as if the words move directly from your heart through the pen and onto the paper, as if your conscious mind is not involved in the process. That's good! This flow can be the entry into an uncharted insight or connection you've never noticed before—the beginning of the new Story of Your Life.

Silence the censor

Do your best to not censor or edit yourself. Just write whatever comes out. If you can't think of a particular word, use another word, or draw a line instead, like this: _____. You can fill in the blank later.

Be kind and keep going

Be kind to yourself. Don't judge yourself or your writing. Whatever you journal is simply an expression of what you're feeling or thinking *at that moment*. It's not written in stone, and you can always change your mind later. Sometimes the words will flow out of you; other times they will need a push (which is when you should keep your pen moving anyway). Whatever the case, *keep going*. Journaling gets easier the more you practice it.

Use your prompts

In this book, you'll most often use what's called a "prompt," a phrase to get your writing started. You begin with the prompt, then take off from there. Some prompts will get your juices flowing while others won't. That's to be expected. If you start writing from a prompt and it doesn't work for you, you can write something else, but at least try writing from the prompt first. And if you begin with the prompt, but the writing takes you in a new direction, that's fine. Go with the flow of your thoughts, wherever it takes you. Sometimes one prompt will be similar to another close by, but both are meant to help you explore the same topic from a slightly different angle.

Do what you can

Not everyone who uses this book will be able to write for each exercise or each prompt. Your ability and desire will depend on the type and extent of your injury and other factors. Just do the exercises you are capable of doing. Over time, you may be able to do more.

Just write

Most of the exercises also allow for a journal entry that does not begin with a prompt. Look for "Freewrite" when you want to write about the topic without the structure of a prompt. Furthermore, if you ever want to journal without this book, you can use a prompt if you have one, but know that it's not necessary. Just begin to write about whatever is on your mind.

Skipping prompts

If a prompt makes you uncomfortable or nervous, feel free to skip it. However, consider three things before you decide. First, no one else ever has to see your writing, so you can be as personal and open as you want. Second, if you can manage to write about something that frightens you or makes you nervous, your uneasiness may slowly dissolve. Third—this is the most important consideration—respect your feelings when you *really don't* want to pursue a topic you find painful or frightening. The purpose here is not to force yourself to write about difficult subjects, but to realize how far you want to venture at this point in your journey. If you don't want to use a particular prompt one day, know that you'll probably feel more comfortable using it another time. And if you have a counselor or therapist, please discuss the prompts that make you uneasy.

Start the journey

Remember: After you write in your journal, you will be a different person than before you wrote, if only in the tiniest way. You reached inside and experienced something new within yourself. You put your thoughts on paper and created a new story, even if it was only a few sentences long. Sometimes that little seed is the first step in a wonderful, exciting journey.

Group Journaling

Journal writing is usually a solitary activity, yet journaling with others can offer companionship and social contact—both important concerns for people with brain injury. The authors have led journal groups for people with brain injury for several years. In our groups of four to six participants, we begin with an explanation of the first topic for the day, and then everyone writes from the same prompt. We normally cover two or three prompts in a 90-minute session. After each writing, those who wish can read their journal entry to the group. This reading aloud is absolutely voluntary; no one is ever pressured to do so.

We have only two rules for our groups. If you decide to form a journal group, please follow them. Remember:

Rule 1: Listen to one another with respect.

Don't judge other people or what they have written. Everyone in the group has his or her own story, and it's not your job to judge them in a negative way, although people often appreciate supportive comments. A journal group should be a safe place. If people make negative comments about each other, that safety will disappear.

Rule 2: What happens in the group stays in the group.

Everything revealed there is confidential and should not be discussed outside the group with anyone else.

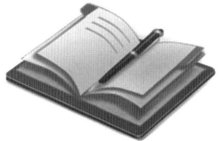

Relax Before a Journaling Session

A good way to begin a journaling session is to relax and release the cares of your day. This will quiet your mind and help you focus on the writing.

- Play quiet, soothing instrumental music if you like.
- Sit comfortably in your chair, feet on the floor and hands on your lap.
- Close your eyes and pay attention to your breath as you breathe slowly, in…and…out, in…and…out.
- Feel yourself sink into the chair.
- Use your slow breathing to relax further into your body.
- Let the tensions and concerns of the day flow out and away.
- If tensions come back, let them flow away again. If they remain, that's fine. Simply accept their presence without stress.
- Know you are in a safe, comfortable place.
- Know that whatever you write will be helpful to you.
- Continue to relax and breathe slowly for at least three to five minutes.
- Gradually open your eyes and gently come back to awareness.
- If you are playing music, you can let it continue or turn it off. If you leave it on while you journal, remember that music can affect your mood.

On some days you may be angry or frustrated. You might want nothing more than to vent in your journal. When that happens, feel free to plunge right into the writing without relaxing first. Let it all out on the page! WRITE BIG if it feels good. Who says you have to write on the lines? Ignore the lines and scribble away! Chances are, the act of writing will reduce or release the upset you're feeling, and you might even find a solution to the problem. Remember, this is *your* journal and you are writing pieces of *your* story.

In the following pages, you will find journaling topics divided into the following chapters, each containing exercises with a variety of prompts:

Chapter 1   After Brain Injury: What Happened? What Can I Discover?
Chapter 2   Loss and Change: Brain Power, Memory, and More
Chapter 3   Relationships: Family, Friends, and Others
Chapter 4   Adjustments: Anger and Grief

Chapter 5   Back Into the Community: Moving Forward With Hope

Chapter 6   Later On: Any Positives?

Chapter 7   Miscellaneous Prompts

The exercises in this workbook are labeled "My Story," and they are numbered according to the order in which they appear in the chapters, for easy reference. Each exercise generally has several prompts. For instance, "My Story 1-1" is Chapter 1, first exercise, and "My Story 5-4" is Chapter 5, fourth exercise.

Recap

When you journal, it is *your* time for *your* writing. With this book, you can move in order through the topics and prompts or you can jump around, choosing whichever one feels right at the moment. You can use each exercise numerous times or only once or never (although we hope you try them all). Remember that no matter how many times you write from the same prompt, you're likely to discover new insights or alternate ways of looking at the situation each time you choose it. You can journal once a day or several times a week, or whenever the mood strikes and time allows. Having a regular journal practice allows you to track your progress, especially as you move through difficult periods in your life.

To use this book you will need a separate journal. You can begin with the lined pages at the back of this book. There are many beautiful journals available today—just be sure to choose one that's comfortable to use and easy to write in. You can also use a three-ring binder and add pages as necessary, or use a plain spiral notebook. Whenever you journal, write the date and the prompt at the top of the page and take off from there. By dating your entries, you can follow the pattern of your thoughts over time.

- Each time you journal, remember:
- Keep your pen moving for the whole time if at all possible.
- If you get stuck, write "I am stuck" or keep repeating the last few words until the flow begins again.
- Go with the flow of your thoughts—don't think or plan ahead about what you will write.
- Do your best not to judge or censor yourself or the words on the page.
- Give yourself wholehearted permission to write whatever you want to write, and then do it.

If you like, begin with a short time of relaxation.

After that, if you have a timer or an alarm, set it for however long you want to write, say 10 or 20 minutes, so you will not have to interrupt the flow of your writing to check the time. Then pick up your pen or go to your computer or recording device and begin.

Chapter 1
After Brain Injury: What Happened? What Can I Discover?

"Writing makes a map, and there is something about a journey that begs to have its passage marked."
Christina Baldwin
Life's Companion: Journal Writing as a Spiritual Practice

If you are using this book to tell the story of your brain injury and its effects on your life, you are seeking to make sense of what has happened. Congratulations for choosing to describe your journey! You have taken a courageous step.

Whatever its cause—such as a vehicle crash, fall, sports injury, tumor, illness, exposure to a blast, violence, or surgery—each brain injury is as unique as the person to whom it happens. Since the brain is intimately involved in everything we do, a brain injury can affect not only physical functions but also those behaviors and cognitive abilities that make us who we are. Physically, a brain injury can alter vision, hearing, taste, smell, touch, or mobility, for example. On the cognitive and behavioral side, a brain injury can affect personality, memory, the ability to learn and concentrate, self-control, motivation, and more. Any one of these changes—let alone several—can throw a life out of its familiar patterns, causing confusion, stress, and worse.

Your doctors, therapists, and other resources can give you a great deal of information about your injury and what you may expect. At the same time, you know yourself much better than anyone. Minute by minute, you experience your life, including what is happening to you as a result of the injury, even if you cannot yet put it into words. With these journaling exercises, you will be able to explore yourself and your life to gain some helpful insights. You will learn more about yourself each time you write.

In this section, you will begin your journey by writing about your brain injury and your brain. Remember to do your relaxation technique on page 10 before you begin if you like.

My Story 1-1
How My Injury Happened

→ Begin with relaxation technique. Refer to page 10.

Your brain injury happened as a result of an event or a situation. To begin telling your story in this journal, begin by writing about that event or situation. Write as much as you can in the time you have set.

```
    I remember clearly…. We had just finished lunch and I was
instructing. The class was practicing in the river bales, a
setting much like a gazebo. These did not have railings (I had
asked for railings and I had asked for one less table on this
bale because it made it tight for the therapist to walk around
the massage tables).
    One of the students needed assistance and I started to her aid
suddenly I had the feeling that the floor slid away from me. I
had my fingers on a support pillar and it felt as if it moved
away from me, too…it was a surreal feeling. And, then I realized
there was air under my feet. Six meters of air before I would
land on concrete or water. I was hoping for water, I got both!...
    My head hit a concrete flower pot that cracked open, and I
thought, 'that is not good', sure that it was my head that
cracked open…Fear was starting to take over my body. I truly felt
my head was cracked open, my neck was in pain, and I felt as if
my brain was swelling, and blood was everywhere. - **Lela**
```

Choose one of these prompts:

Date: _____
- ☞ If you remember the event or situation that caused your brain injury, use this:
- ✎ I remember that my brain injury happened…

- ☞ OR, if you are unable to remember the event or situation that caused your brain injury, and it was explained to you later, use this:
- ✎ As I was told later, my brain injury happened when…

- ✎ Freewrite...

My Story 1-2
How It Feels to be Me

After a brain injury, you're very likely to feel different in some ways than you felt before it happened. How do you feel different? How do you feel the same? (Since it is probable that you will feel different in some way every day, this is a good prompt to use often.)

```
This is how it feels to be me today: I got pushed into a room
with no windows and somebody broke the lightbulbs and slammed the
door. There is nothing all around me. Once in a while, the door
opens a crack and I see out but not much. How could a little fall
do this to me. - Andy

Getting hit in the head makes things harder. - Nathan
```

Choose one of these prompts:

Date: _____
- ✎ This is how it feels to be me today...

- ☞ Next, if you don't like the way you're feeling, write about how you would like to feel instead. It is sometimes possible to improve your mood and perhaps even your physical state by actively thinking yourself into a better one.

- ✎ I wish I could feel this way instead...
- ✎ Freewrite...

My Story 1-3
The Worst Part

After undergoing a trauma, many people find it difficult to explain or explore the worst parts of the experience, even to themselves. They may feel confused or frightened about what happened, embarrassed or ashamed (even though the event might not have been their fault), or they may simply not know how to begin. If you're up to it and can give yourself permission to explore the worst part of your injury, try these next prompts.

☞ The "worst part" can be the physical damage to the brain itself, the cause of the injury, a negative change in your life, or anything else that might have happened. If you're hesitant to work with this prompt, remember that no one else has to see what you write. In addition, the wording of the first prompt, with "If I could tell the story," lets you slide into the writing rather than confront it head on.

If you're already comfortable writing about this issue, choose the second prompt.

Remember, if you're working with a counselor or therapist, you can discuss this exercise before or after you try it, if that will help you feel safer or more comfortable with it.

Date: _____
- ✏ If I could tell the story about the worst part of my brain injury, I would say…
- ✏ The worst part of my brain injury…
- ✏ Freewrite…

16 After Brain Injury: Telling Your Story

My Story 1-4
Making Metaphor

A metaphor* is a figure of speech in which one thing is referred to as another. For instance, "my baby is a gorgeous flower" describes the baby's beauty by comparing her to a flower, and "the black puddle of cat sleeping on the floor" is a colorful way of describing how the curled-up cat appears to the viewer.

Our brains seem to be hardwired to respond to metaphors (it may be harder to recognize them after a brain injury). We use them frequently and don't even realize it. For instance, if someone is a pest, we call the person "a pain in the neck." If someone is emotionally strong, we say he or she is "a rock." Some other common and often unrealized metaphors: time is money; in over my head; or love is "up" and sadness is "down." Metaphors can also be extended, as in these examples.

```
My motorcycle accident was on 28 September 2007. I tell people
that each day it's like as if you went to bed and you woke up in
China or New York City not knowing how you got there. It's like I
don't speak the same language as everyone else anymore. Not
knowing how you ended up in this strange place is how I feel all
the time. - Michael

Before my brain injury, my memory was like a long shelf that
could hold a lot. Now, it's much shorter, and memories fall off
the back when I add new ones to the front. - Ken
```

Metaphors can add an emotional punch to a description, as these statements show. Upon reading them, you can sense that Michael's awakening from a coma was like waking up in a world entirely unfamiliar and strange to him, and how he still feels he doesn't fit in. Ken's metaphor uses a visual image to describe how his memory, which cannot be seen, works now.

Try your hand at creating metaphors about brain injury. To do this, think about how it feels physically or emotionally to have a brain injury. Then see if your imagination or spirit of creativity can compare it to something else. Creating some metaphors about brain injury might help you—and others—better understand what you are going through. If you say, "Having a brain injury is like living in a puzzle where some of the pieces are missing," people will immediately understand your meaning. Here's another example: "Since my brain injury, I can focus about as well as a hummingbird," which means you can rarely stay focused but instead flit from one activity or thought to another.

☞ You can start with the prompts below or begin in any way that works for you:

Date: _____
- A brain injury is like…
- Living with a brain injury is…
- A brain injury is as…
- Having a brain injury…
- Freewrite...

*For the gramatically-minded: A comparison containing the words "like" or "as" is called a simile. For ease of understanding we used "metaphor" to include both terms.

My Story 1-5
Talking with Your Brain

In this two-part entry, you will look into your brain and then talk with it. It's fascinating territory! But don't worry—you don't need a microscope or an MRI or any medical background. You need only your imagination and some crayons or colored markers.

Begin with the drawing of the human brain below. First, use your imagination to "listen" to what it is saying to you. Next, use your crayons or markers to decorate it however you like. You don't need to be an artist. Your imagination will guide you, so go with the flow.

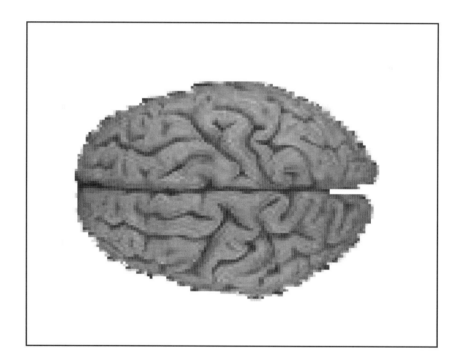

Now that you have symbolically entered your brain, write a dialogue with it, as you would a script for a movie or a play. You will write both your words and what you imagine your brain is saying in response, as if it were another person. Sure, you're making up both sides of the dialogue, but that's what makes this such an interesting process.

If writing a dialogue feels uncomfortable at first, know that it will become more comfortable as you practice. If you feel silly because you're "talking to yourself" (and truly, that is what you're doing), give yourself permission to feel silly, knowing that you are using a creative tool to learn more about your inner self. (Besides, no one else ever has to see it.) Dialogue is a directed process that often allows insights to arise—some of which may surprise you. You can dialogue with anything or anybody, real or imagined, since you "play" both parts.

Our bodies possess an innate wisdom, and by using dialogue, we can often allow that wisdom to come to the surface. After an illness or injury, a dialogue with the affected body parts can bring to light the hidden elements, those things that have not yet revealed themselves, and perhaps begin the journey to restoration and healing.

B: [Brain]: R u awake?
M: [Me]: Ya, why?
B: I wanted to remind u that I'm still here & fully functional.
M: What do u mean?
B: Just because we were injured, we're not destroded [destroyed].
M: What do we know?
B: Rebuild my connection & knowledge.
M: How?
B: What r the positive, outcomes do u want with yr life?
M: There's a lot.
B: Well, concentrate on those positive aspects & believe in them & tell them me to them every day.
M: OK, I will.
B: Thoughts r powerful tools. – **Todd**, May 2008

   Me: Now that you and I can see and understand some other people, isn't it unbelievable how many others are stuck inside themselves. Why?
   Brain: Well, there's multipal levels to me functioning and it seems they are stuck inside themselves because they question themselves on how and why to act so other people will think better of them or like them better. Instead of them liking and loving themselves for who they are and what they can achieve.
   Me: It's almost as if they're lieing to themselves.
   Brain: Yes, and they've not had a brain injury. – **Todd**, September 2008

☞ If you want a starting point, here are some to choose from:

✎ Dialogue with your brain about how it or you have changed since it was injured.

✎ Ask your brain questions, perhaps about how it works now or what it feels like to be an injured brain.

✎ Tell your brain something you would like it to know, and see what it says in response.

Date: _____
✎ For your dialogue with your brain, write as many lines for "Me" and "Brain" as necessary...
Me:
Brain:

✎ Freewrite...

After Brain Injury: Telling Your Story

My Story 1-6
Map to My True Self

Even though you've undergone some changes—possibly even major ones—because of the injury to your brain, your True Self has not changed. This deepest part of you cannot be affected by outside forces. Some people call the True Self the spirit or soul or life force; others consider it to be the basic energy from which all things are created. You might call it something else. Whatever its name, it is like an enduring flame that never flickers out. It exists within you simply because you exist. What's more, you can call on your True Self for courage, patience, and the ability to continue on, no matter what's happening around you or to you.

How would you define your True Self? Do you think your memories and personality play a role in it? Do you think it goes deeper than that? Do you feel it might have changed after your injury? And how do you find it or communicate with it?

☞ This journaling exercise has two parts. For the first part, you'll need crayons or colored markers to draw a "Map to My True Self" in whatever way you feel moved or inspired to do that. Don't worry that you have to be an artist—not at all! You can add whatever elements your imagination creates to lead you to it. Whatever form it takes on the page is perfect, so let yourself enjoy the experience. The second part will be a journal entry as usual.

☞ Before you begin drawing, relax for a few minutes. Sit comfortably in your chair, feet on the floor and hands on your lap. Close your eyes and pay attention to your breath as you breathe slowly in and out. Feel your body sink into the chair, then relax into your body with your slow breathing. Feel the tensions and concerns of the day flow out and away. Know that this is a safe, comfortable place, and the drawing and writing you do will be helpful. As you continue to breathe slowly and relax, ask your True Self to reveal itself so that you can draw a path to it. It is present within you and will feel honored by your request.

☞ Then draw your Map to My True Self in your journal or notebook. Take as long as you like. After your map feels complete, use this prompt.

Date: _____

✎ After drawing my Map to My True Self, I know this thing I didn't know before…

My Story 1-7
Kindred Spirits, or Not

After sustaining a brain injury, the resulting confusion and unexpected life changes can leave you feeling lost. One way to begin finding your way back to a feeling of security and wholeness is to find kindred spirits—characters you identify with—and journal about them. These characters can be real people in your life, or they can come from books, movies, or television. They can be animals, such as your dog that loves you enthusiastically or a fierce bear that fears nothing. They can come directly from your imagination. Whoever or whatever they are, your kindred spirits have a trait or a quality you would like to possess, such as inner strength or compassion or a sense of humor.

Some days you might not want to write about a kindred spirit. You might instead feel like writing about a character with qualities you do *not* want to keep or develop, such as being in denial or projecting nothing but gloom and doom. At those times you can journal about why you prefer not to be like that—unless of course you see their qualities as valuable in your current stage of recovery and want to explore them in yourself.

> I think I identify with the Little Engine That Could. I've been in 3 major wrecks in this life and have fought back from all of them to a place beyond the prognosis. The only saving factor for me was just because I was at the wrong place at exactly the right time. I was never the direct cause, just a direct participant. I never really considered giving up and staying broken. Every little improvement gave me hope that something else could happen that would again show me that I was moving forward. I will keep working to get over the hills I keep putting in my path. - **Phil**

With this exercise, you might discover some element of yourself you can learn to depend on in the days ahead. You might also discover an inner area you would like to strengthen so you can better support yourself. And should you feel not very cheerful or positive, putting those feelings down on paper may help release those feelings. Remember, journaling is an opportunity to write about *whatever* you're experiencing, and you can keep your writing private if you so choose. Being as honest as you can in your writing is healthier than hiding those things you believe might be unacceptable or negative. It takes a lot of energy to hide from yourself, energy you could be using for healing and recovery.

☞ Give yourself permission to write *whatever* you feel as you journal. And remember, if you are working with a counselor or therapist, feel free to share your writing in a session.

Date: _____
- ____(Name)____ is a kindred spirit to me because…
- I identify with...
- I do NOT want to be a kindred spirit with ____(Name)____ because…
- Freewrite...

My Story 1-8
What Else Happened to Me?

So far in this section, you've explored your brain, dialogued with it, and investigated various aspects of your brain injury. Now you can use what you've discovered to move your exploration one step further.

In addition to the actual cause of your brain injury, many other things happened to you as a result. You and your life were changed in some ways. Perhaps you are already able to make a list of those changes. Or even with a list, you might not feel emotionally ready to explore them. On the other hand, maybe you can't yet name or list them, although you can sense their presence.

```
    Am I with such adynamia that I am not able to see, understand
in what state of action-less, wordless, look-less condition I am
in. I am aware that it is difficult to stay focused on a subject
or action when I am the only one around, which is about 95% of my
time. I do enjoy other people's energy and it helps give me a
direction. Is that 95% of voided time working against my recovery,
throwing me deeper into a hill climb out of this confusion of a
head injury? I do have thoughts that run through my broken mind,
mostly pictures. When I try to share those thoughts with another,
picking the correct words, looking through my mind to find the
correct words, to get those words to speak out of my mouth, then
not know for sure the words I am speaking are the ones I have
found. Quite often, they are not the words I found. Some of the
words are similar to the words I found in my mind maze, other
words are nowhere close and make no sense. - **Todd**
```

☞ If you can name or list some of the results of what happened to you that day, go right to the next prompt and start writing. But if you haven't yet been able to figure out what they are, use your relaxation technique and ask these changes to gently reveal themselves to you. Then when you are ready, go to the next prompt and begin writing. If you write from this prompt every so often, you'll be able to name additional changes that have happened as a result of the injury.

➜ Begin with relaxation technique. Refer to page 10.

Date: _____

✎ In your journal, make a list of other things that happened to you as a result of your injury. Write the numbers 1 - 10. Fill in as many as you can.

✎ Something else that happened to me that day was…
✎ If I was able to name something else that happened to me that day, it would be…
✎ Freewrite...

22 After Brain Injury: Telling Your Story

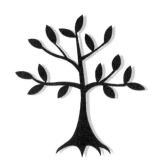

Chapter 2
Loss and Change:
Brain Power, Memory, and More

*"Stories are medicine, small doses of what matters, and it is the telling
that releases the medicine, the telling that soothes our pain and shares our joy…."*
Mark Nepo, *The Exquisite Risk*

"God gave us memory so that we might have roses in December."
J.M. Barrie, Scottish novelist

Your brain injury might have happened in an instant, as with a fall, a vehicle crash, or an explosion. It might have taken place over time, from a brain tumor or an infection in the brain. Yet regardless of how long it took, you were changed and your life was altered. These changes can be small or enormous. They can be short-lived or permanent. Sometimes they can be overcome, other times not. In general, a brain injury causes loss of some kind, and that can be devastating.

You might have lost:

- ✓ physical abilities such as vision, hearing, sense of smell, balance, coordination, speech, swallowing, or muscle function;
- ✓ cognitive abilities such as memory, the ability to concentrate or organize, mental processing speed, the ability to read and write, word recall and language, or various perceptual skills;
- ✓ social or behavioral abilities such as the ability to monitor your behavior or language, the ability to cope or relate to others, motivation, creativity, or self-esteem; or
- ✓ your job or place in school, your marriage or other important relationships, financial security, or your driver's license.

Because of the losses, you also might have lost your sense of self, those qualities and elements that make you YOU. Included here could be things you cannot name or cannot quite identify, but which you sense are missing and know are important to you.

It's common and natural for survivors to grieve the loss of "who I used to be" when they cannot function the way they did before the brain injury. Fortunately for many survivors, some losses can be restored over time, at least partially. If survivors are able to gain enough awareness of their situation, they may be able to accept it, which can in turn enable them to build new skills or compensate for or accommodate what has been lost.

☞ Following are some prompts you can use when writing about loss.

My Story 2-1
Loss List

☞ Consider what you have lost because of your brain injury and make a Loss List in your journal. Write the numbers 1-10. Fill in as many as you can.

Date: _____

✎ Loss List...

```
1.  independence
2.  boyfriend
3.  cheerleader
4.  basketball scholarship
5.  grades in school
6.  senior prom
7.  driving
8.  normal use of arm
9.  weekend job
    - Steph
```

✎ Freewrite:

My Story 2-2
Empty Spaces

Can you remember a time when you lost something important to you? Maybe as a child you had a beloved doll or toy you turned to for comfort, and one day you could not find it anywhere. Or perhaps, later in life, you lost a cherished piece of jewelry that had been given to you by someone you loved. There are other kinds of losses, too, such as divorce or the end of a friendship, getting fired or laid off from your job, or losing your health to a serious illness. Any of these losses can leave an empty space in your life and in your heart. So can a brain injury.

```
    The brain injury has left me with an empty space that used to
be filled with a certainty about who I was and what I strived to
achieve, a lovingly dysfunctional family, tons of friends,
professional friends/colleagues, fulfilling & challenging work,
students, the ability to constantly learn new things, a body in
excellent physical condition, laughter, joy, fun, the means to
pursue my passions (reading, writing, painting, traveling (6/7
times/year), athletics, managing, teaching, debating, and music).
```
– Kirsten

☞ Choose one of these prompts to write about either an item from your Loss List or another loss:

Date: _____
- ✎ The brain injury has left me with an empty space that used to be filled with…
- ✎ Something I can no longer do because of the brain injury is _____
- ✎ Freewrite...

My Story 2-3
Unnamed Losses

It's very possible you may have suffered losses you cannot really put your finger on. Deep down, you know that something important has disappeared or changed drastically, but you don't know what to call it. This feeling of uncertainty can make you uneasy or jumpy. It might frustrate you because if you knew what it was, you could deal with it. Would you like to try?

You might be able to name or describe this loss by responding to the next journaling prompt. But first, close your eyes, sit quietly, and relax as you have been doing for some of the prompts.

➜ Begin with relaxation technique. Refer to page 10.

As you relax your body, do your best to let your mind and emotions relax as well. Let your cares flow away. Don't struggle to find a name or description for this loss. Instead, as you continue to breathe slowly in and out, in and out, ask this unnamed loss to reveal itself. Then notice how you feel in your body. Does part of your body hurt or tingle or feel somehow different? That might be a clue. Can you sense something stirring in your heart or your spirit? That's another clue.

If you don't experience any physical feelings or stirrings, that's fine, too. Continue to sit and relax for 5 or 10 minutes more. When you're ready, pick up your pen and begin writing whatever comes to mind. Don't judge your writing or try to censor it. Just let it flow and see what happens. You can always come back to this prompt any time and try again.

Date:_____
- ✎ The nameless thing I have lost now has a name, which is _____. I can now begin to deal with it because…
- ✎ The nameless thing I have lost now has a name, which is _____. I am not yet ready to deal with it because…
- ✎ Freewrite...

My Story 2-4
Glued Together

In one of his poems, Rainer Marie Rilke used this phrase: "…right there I am sort of glued together." That's a wonderful metaphor that can be interpreted in different ways. Sometimes, gluing things together makes them stronger, as when a woodworker glues two pieces of wood in addition to using nails or another method of joining. Yet sometimes when a broken thing is glued back together, the stuck-together pieces are never again as strong as the whole object used to be.

Do you feel now as if the brain injury left you broken and then the pieces were glued together, but not quite the right way? Are there now pieces missing, leaving gaps? Maybe you feel jagged or wobbly, like a vase that has been poorly put back together.

On the other hand, perhaps you feel that you were "glued together" better than you were before the injury, at least in some ways. Maybe you feel stronger or better able to cope with changes in your life. Perhaps you don't feel glued together at all. Perhaps you still feel whole.

```
They didn't do a very good job gluing me back together
because, well, I have to ask, they who? What's the glue? Is it a
solid glue or pliable glue, elastic? What parts are glued? Are
there different types of glue for different applications?
Physical, mental & emotion? How do I know if the glue parts are
put back together with the right/correct parts? Glue only works
when compatible parts are available to be aplyed to. Am I glued
good? Still working on that question. - Todd

I am stronger now than ever because even though I leak emotion
I am stronger. I've developed a thick skin where they went in and
out twice before and patched me back together. The skull bone has
thickened and been reinforced with titanium mesh and a few loose
screws. The "dura matter" thickened to protect me. So now I can
really say I am one "tough mother." - Anne
```

☞ Try one of these prompts to explore this feeling of "…right there I am sort of glued together":

Date: _____
- The place where I am glued together is...
- They didn't do a very good job gluing me back together because...
- I am stronger now than ever because...
- What I wish could have been glued together better is...
- Freewrite...

After Brain Injury: Telling Your Story

My Story 2-5
Off Balance

Any kind of shock or trauma can throw a life emotionally off-balance. With a brain injury, the physical ability to balance can also be affected. Either way, it feels uncomfortable and sometimes even dangerous. For those times when you feel off-balance in any way, use these prompts.

```
    To regain my balance, I need more money. I need more loving
acceptance of my processing methods. Life is a process and self-
reflection and self-examination are essential parts of the whole.
I'm very proud of my lifelong activities as a student and
volunteer. I just don't have all the degress and letters/popular
acclaim. The natural world of growing things, plants and animals.
Others need to stop trying to control my individual choices about
smoking and off-label drug use [to control a brain tumor]. I have
regained my balance - focus from others. -
```
Anne

Date: _____
- 🖉 To regain my balance, I need…
- 🖉 Something that pushes me off-balance is…
- 🖉 People could help me keep my balance if…
- 🖉 I'm staying balanced by…
- 🖉 Freewrite...

My Story 2-6
Memory

Tennessee Williams, the playwright, wrote, "Life is all memory, except for that one present moment that goes by you so quickly, you hardly catch it going." Memory allows you to benefit not only from knowledge you have accumulated on your own, but also from knowledge earlier generations possessed and passed on—everything from how to plant crops or build a house, to brushing your teeth and driving. It also allows you to form connections with others and with events, which provides a sense of belonging and of continuity over time.

Memory loss is one of the most common cognitive results of brain injury, even with mild ones. There are three major types of memory that will be explored here—immediate, short-term, and long-term. Survivors of brain injury can have deficits in one or all of them.

Immediate memory holds short bits of information for a few seconds or minutes. An example: calling 411 to get a phone number, hearing the number, and then being able to call it without writing it down. People with damage to immediate memory might be asked to do a task, agree to do it, and within a few seconds, forget the entire episode. They might put down their eyeglasses or keys and instantly have no memory of where they left them. They can walk into a room with absolutely no recall about why they did so, or turn to the refrigerator with the intent of taking out a particular item but forget which one by the time they have opened the door.

Short-term memory is also known as recent memory or new learning. It holds the information you need to remember in the following minutes, hours, or days. Short-term memory loss can take many forms. For instance, someone with a brain injury might be able to read a short story but cannot recall it later that day. Another survivor might easily recall old friends when they come to visit (good long-term memory), but ten minutes afterward have no memory of them being in the room. Another might be able to make appointments for the upcoming week but then cannot remember them.

Long-term memory is information that can be recalled days, months, or years later. This is someone's general fund of knowledge, much of it gathered before the brain injury. It includes such items as one's name and the names of family and friends, one's address and phone number, schools attended, favorite childhood vacation, and for people in the United States, the number of states or the name of the first U.S. president.

```
    A particularly difficult memory came when I was working. I
had a job at a dude ranch which played nothing but country
western radio, yet one day, on the station due to a request, the
song "The First Time" by Roberta Flack played. In college, a
dozen years before, I had been engaged to an amazing man who died
tragically in a car accident two months before the wedding. That
was our song, as it was playing the first time he saw me at a
school dance. I was standing near a light which seemed to put a
halo by shining through my hair and he told his roommate "I am
going to marry that woman." After a few months of him chasing me
I finally agreed to date. I was very shy but after two years I
agreed to marriage. Yet he died, knocking me off track. At the
age of twenty-one, death is not an option.
```

> So there I stood, listening to a song and sobbing for an unknown reason. I had to leave the front office and go into my own, my head spinning. Still, I did not remember. Two days later, the same song played on the same country western station and I broke down again, but this time the memories flood through, only they felt as fresh as the day I picked up a telephone to hear a friend say, "Lesley, I need to tell your something. Please sit down…" – **Lesley**

Memory may not be as accurate or as strong as it was before the injury. Some survivors can easily remember their lives up until the injury, but afterward they have difficulty forming new memories. Less often, they might forget large chunks of their pre-injury memories. Their memory loss might be more selective in that they may find it difficult to remember how to do simple, everyday tasks. They may remember procedures very well but have problems with formulating and remembering concepts.

> When you don't have a cast or big bandages people think you are normal. My mother died in 1992 on my 32nd birthday of cancer. My wife told me that I was all ways wondering and asking her and my father how come my mom hasn't visited me yet at the hospital. That's how badly my memory was affected. – **Michael**

Human beings create the story of their lives from the memories they make. It has been said that humans are their memories. So how do they cope when they can no longer remember, or remember well? When amnesia wipes out some old memories, or deficits in short-term memory make it challenging to retain new memories, what happens to their story, and to their life? A serious memory loss truly can be considered a major loss of self, and even a slight memory deficiency can cause immense problems for a survivor.

☞ If you have a memory loss of some kind from your injury, try some of the following prompts:

Date: _____
- When I forget something I think I should remember, I…
- What others don't understand about my memory now is…
- The worst thing about my memory loss is…
- If I could remember one thing I've forgotten, it would be…
- To cope with my memory loss, I've learned to…
- People finish my sentences for me now, and that makes me…
- I know how to drive, but they tell me I can't, and…
- Freewrite...

My Story 2-7
Memory Lists

This is an exercise you can use often to challenge your memory. Simply jot down 10 memories as they come to mind. They can be people, places, objects, events, or anything else that pops up. They can be important, like your wedding, or not, like the glazed doughnut you had for breakfast. If your memory now works at a slower pace, give yourself all the time you need. You can even write a few items on the list, stop, and then come back to it later. However, if you want to challenge yourself, you can set a timer to see if you can complete the list before the buzzer goes off.

Date: _____
✎ As quickly as you can, list 10 items in your journal that you remember from *before* your injury.

Date: _____
✎ As quickly as you can, list 10 items in your journal you remember from *after* your injury.

Once you complete a list, you can choose an item and journal about it for a few minutes. (Also see "Using the Senses to Remember," My Story 2-13, Chapter 2, for a longer memory exercise.) You can use one of these prompts or start writing on your own.

Date: _____
✎ An old memory I love is…
✎ A recent memory I love is…
✎ Freewrite...

After Brain Injury: Telling Your Story 31

My Story 2-8
Improving Memory

People with brain injuries who have memory loss can often boost their memory's ability. Some take notes or use a recording device; this serves as an ongoing kind of memory book. Sometimes brain training exercises can help strengthen memory "muscle." What have you been able to do to improve your memory's function?

☞ Use your personal experience to think about your memory.

Date: _____
✎ Some strategies I've developed to help me remember are…
✎ I have made progress with improving my memory by…
✎ Something happened to show me that my memory is improving, and…
✎ Freewrite…

My Story 2-9
Other Functions Lost

In addition to harming memory, a brain injury can disrupt other mental functions. For instance, a common problem for survivors is word recall, also called the "tip of the tongue phenomenon." They may well know the word they want to use and may even be able to visualize a picture of it in their mind's eye, but they cannot retrieve it from their brain's language center. This can make it extremely difficult to carry on a conversation or to write.

> I got so frustrated when I knew what I wanted to say but couldn't pull up the right words. They just wouldn't come to me. When I came home from rehab, I knew I had trimmed the trees in our backyard and cleared out something from the branches right before the accident. I could see a picture of it in my mind, but all that I could say to describe it was "Christmas kissing stuff." My wife told me the word was "mistletoe," and instantly I knew that was right. Five years later, this still happens, but it's not as bad. – **Ken**

A number of physical functions and abilities can also be affected by brain injury, altering the survivor's life in many ways.

> Because some parts of my body don't work as well as they did, it takes me so much longer to get around now. I am walking and I'm happy about that but my leg doesn't move the same any more and it takes so much more focus just to move about the house let alone out of the house. – **Shannon**

☞ Look at the prompts below to see which ones you might want to include in your journaling about losses. Over time, try all those that fit your situation.

Date: _____
- When I can't think of the word, it would help me if people would…
- What I want to say is on the tip of my tongue, but…
- Living in my body now feels like…
- Because some parts of my body don't work as well as they did…
- The most bothersome thing about the physical changes I've experienced is…
- My mind used to be _____ and now it is…
- It used to be so easy to _____ but now it's much harder because…
- The most important thing I lost is…
- I used to be _____ and now I am…
- I had lost _____ after the brain injury, but it is returning, and…
- Freewrite…

After Brain Injury: Telling Your Story 33

My Story 2-10
Because of These Losses

Sadly, many people with brain injury suffer other losses because of their physical and mental changes. The list can include divorce, broken friendships, a changed relationship with children or family, formerly good health, or not being able to return to work or school or having to return in a lesser capacity. They may no longer be able to enjoy favorite activities such as sports, playing a musical instrument, reading, and so on. Because of all the changes, the "old me"—or large portions of it—can disappear.

☞ Use these prompts below to explore other losses due to brain injury:

Date: _____
- The biggest thing now lost from my life is _____ and that feels…
- I wish I could still _____ because…
- The brain injury affected the "old me" by…
- The part of the "old me" I miss the most is _____ because…
- Now that certain functions or abilities are lost to me, I don't feel worthy of…
- With all these losses, I'm afraid of…
- No one can relate to what I'm going through because…
- Freewrite...

34 After Brain Injury: Telling Your Story

My Story 2-11
Resilience

"Barn's burnt down… Now I can see the moon."

This simple declaration was expressed by the 17th-century Japanese poet Masahide, after his barn actually did go up in flames. In addition to being eloquent, it is a wonderful statement of the quality of resilience, or the psychological ability to cope with catastrophe and great stress—and perhaps even to thrive under such conditions. Like Masahide, resilient people tend to bounce back from negative events, make the most of small opportunities, have the emotional wherewithal to cope well with many different situations, are determined to overcome tough challenges, and are able to hang in there during difficult times. In addition, they typically have a supportive network of people to depend on and a strong belief in some system of meaning, such as religion or spirituality or philosophy.

When facing serious trauma or misfortune, resilient people may at first react negatively and may very well feel stressed. However, they are able to find ways to move past that stage and then rebuild or restore their confidence.

Resilience may be inborn in some people, yet many others can develop their "resilience muscles" by training their thoughts, behaviors, and actions. Journaling regularly can improve resilience by recording progress made through a difficult time.

Some ways to develop resilience are:
- ✓ believe that your situation will improve,
- ✓ maintain perspective—don't make mountains out of molehills,
- ✓ take action—even in small ways—to keep moving toward your goals,
- ✓ see how your trauma or challenge has helped you grow in some way, and
- ✓ stay optimistic.

```
    I know I have always been a resilient person because I had to
be. [I was] Born in 1945, [when] my father was in a Belgium
foxhole and when he came home he was a mess. They did not have
psychotherapy for those guys in a small town in Indiana. By the
time I was 6 years old, my mom had married and divorced him 4
times. From the flashbacks and alcohol he was violent, held us at
gun point, burned down our home, and repeatedly abused my mom. So
we moved from Indiana to Alabama. My mom was terrified and took
it all out on me. I had NO support system.
    I still made A's in school. I also had to deal with the
'southern thing' whites against blacks and being a Yankee. I
truly hated Alabama and my mom for taking me there. I wanted to
leave so I packed my bags. I am seven years old. She helped. So
that stopped that. Year after year is another sad childhood
story. I will stop here. I have done my work on those years and I
know that every day prepared me for the rest of my life.
    It is not any different now. Every challenge is truly an
opportunity to see how masterful I can become.
    Out of the many challenges and disappointments and struggling
lifestyle I still landed a good job. Started at 68.00 a week. In
```

```
8 years I was making $30,000, paid vacation, insurance and profit
sharing. I did not go to college. My skills lie in my
organizational ability and attention to detail.
   The funny thing about all of this is I did not plan it. I just
do what is before me and somehow things get done.
   I am doing the same with this injury. Staying aware of my
energy. Doing a little more when my body and brain stem say I
can. Not pushing most of the time. - 
```
Lela

When you have sustained a brain injury and the changes and losses (temporary or permanent) that go with it, you have faced an extremely stressful event. Whether or not you were resilient before your brain injury, remember that you may be able to become resilient now. Ask your counselor or therapist and your social network to help you with this.

```
   Like if you're cut from the team or lose a job, don't curl up
and cry. With a brain injury, you have to keep going. - 
```
Michael

☞ Here are some prompts for writing about resilience:

Date: _____

- I know I have always been a resilient person because…
- My resilience has never been that strong, and I know this because…
- I want to become more resilient, and so I will…
- I know I am quite resilient since my injury because…
- I have overcome many obstacles in my life and…
- I can learn to feel more hopeful about my future by…
- When I'm in a jam, I know I can turn to…
- The people in my life who can help me when I need help…
- I can figure out the difference between things I can change and things that are out of my control by…
- When I know a situation in my life is out of my control, I usually…
- I know that my past difficulties have made me a stronger person because…
- I usually fall apart during difficult times and…
- I am able to learn and grow by…
- When something stressful happens to me, I usually…
- Even in stressful times, I am able to…
- Freewrite...

My Story 2-12
I Still Have This

Even though your brain injury has caused some losses or changes in function, what still works? What has remained? What parts of you or your life still operate well, or maybe even better than they did before?

```
Even though I can't work now, I'm home when my son comes home
from school. He likes that. So do I. — Michael
```

It can take time to realize the positives that can happen after a trauma. Sometimes the positives have to do with simply realizing that the damage could have been worse. Other times, people with brain injury discover that they can still have a good life, even if it is different than their pre-injury life.

☞ Chapter 6 will cover this in more depth, but for now, try some of these prompts:

Date: _____
- Even though some things are gone from my life, I still have…
- There is one part of me that I will never leave behind, and it is…
- Even though my life is more difficult now than before my injury, I can still…
- Something I do now to overcome my fears…
- Freewrite…

After Brain Injury: Telling Your Story 37

My Story 2-13
Using the Senses to Remember

This is a longer, more involved journaling exercise to use your senses to recall memories.

"The senses offer perfect vehicles for writing about our deepest experiences, challenges, issues, memories, and areas that require examination and healing."
Bob Yehling, *Science of Mind*, Oct. 2006

A memory book is a common tool in brain injury rehabilitation, and you have probably used one or are still doing so. It's likely that in the pages of your memory book, you (or someone writing for you) recorded the basic details about what you did each day, such as what you accomplished in your therapy sessions. In that respect, memory books are extremely valuable.

Memories are made in the brain, but everything that becomes a memory first arrives through your senses. Without your ability to taste, touch/feel, see, hear, and smell, you have no way to connect with the world outside your own mind. Your senses give you the raw materials for the stories of your life: the scent of lilies of the valley on a humid summer day, the itchy feel of the sweater your aunt knitted for you, the taste of a hot dog during a ballgame, the sound of a loved one's laughter or a motorcycle's rumble, the sight of black thunderclouds and lightning off in the distance—all these raw materials are neutral until you add meaning to them. And once you add meaning, you begin creating little stories, many of which gather together to become the Big Story that is your life. For instance, that hotdog at the ballpark might represent the first time your dad, who loved baseball, took you to a Major League game, where you both had one of your best outings ever. Even decades later, when you bite into a ballpark hot dog, you may still be able to internally experience the noises, smells, and sights of that day with your dad—even if you are nowhere near a baseball game.

Sometimes your senses can pull up memories without any conscious urging. You might unexpectedly hear a song from your past, and then in your memory you are transported back to the night your crabby grandmother moved in with your family when that same song was playing on the radio in your house. A friend might give you a bouquet of roses and the fragrance reminds you so strongly of the funeral of your childhood best friend that you burst into tears.

Other times, using the senses on purpose to help us remember can improve our memory of specific events or things. It can possibly help our overall memory build more "muscle."

In ancient Greece and Rome, centuries before books or many written materials were easily available, orators were expected to memorize long passages and deliver them without error. They found that an excellent way to remember long blocks of text was to walk around in a familiar place and mentally connect portions of the text with where they moved—at this curve in the path, they memorized that section, or at that grove of trees, they memorized another. They would do this for the entire speech.

Then when they delivered it, they would "walk" through the familiar place in their minds, and those connections allowed them to remember the speech. Today, new research seems to be revealing reasons for why this works. It's called "embodied cognition," or a new model of the mind that shows how we humans use not only our brains but also our entire bodies—including our senses—to think and remember.

A brain injury can affect memory, sometimes dramatically, so this method might not work well, or at all, for you. But you can experiment with it. As an event is happening, make a conscious effort, if possible, to recall the physical sensations you are experiencing. If you can write them down or record them, so much the better. This may reinforce and anchor the event in your memory to better recall it later.

The Place I Remember

With this next exercise, you'll go beyond a basic memory book and use the stories told by your senses to describe a place from your past. This exercise can be enjoyable as well as healing.

First in your journal, make five columns across the top of a page. Label the columns: See - Hear - Taste - Smell - and Touch.

Now, think of a place you remember. It can be important to you, like a favorite vacation spot or the restaurant where you proposed to your future spouse. It can be a place where you spend a lot of time because you have to be there, such as school or work. It can be a location where the memories aren't the most pleasant, but you want to explore your feelings about it. It can be any place that comes to mind, even the room where you are right now.

Next, do your relaxation technique on page 10 again, but with a little twist.

Sit comfortably in your chair, feet on the floor and hands on your lap. Close your eyes and pay attention to your breath as you breathe slowly, in and out. Feel your body sink into the chair, then relax into your body with your slow breathing. Feel the tensions and concerns of the day flow out and away. Know that you are in a safe, comfortable place, and the writing you do will be helpful. As you continue to relax and breathe slowly, remember this place you want to explore with your sense memory. What did you feel, see, hear, smell, and/or taste there? Continue to relax and breathe slowly for 5 to 10 minutes, and do your best to let that place come alive again through your senses.

Now, as best as you can, write down those sensations you remembered in the columns. Try to use simple, concrete words for what you sensed. For the example of going to the ballgame with your dad, some of the words might be: mustard, hot sun, baseball fans applauding or booing, the color of your dad's hair, the red shirt you were wearing, and so on.

Take 5 to 10 minutes for this. Stay as relaxed as possible, so more memories can come up. If you like, put down your pen and relax once more as you sense the place in your memory.

Finally, write about that place, using the sense memories in your list. The concrete words you wrote down will help your feelings come alive as you journal.

Date: _____

✎ The Place I Remember

Sample:

See	Hear	Taste	Smell	Touch
yellow sunshine moving on tent	birds, wind in trees	lollipop	pine needles	laying on blanket
favorite comic book	a light breeze	lemon flavor sucker	ocean air	warm sun on my back
colors of blanket and shadows of branches from the tall trees	squirrels, crows	peanut butter & jelly	peanut butter/jelly	
orange pine needles				
sticky sap				

In this place, I remember, how relaxed I felt lying warm and snug inside the teepee tent. A safe refuge from the stress and strain going on behind me in the house. I could hear the breeze in the tall trees and the birds flitting around outside and above me. The little bossy squirrel who would disturb the peace in the yard by jumping on the bird feeder. I had everything I needed to spend the whole afternoon in my hideout reading my comic books without anyone hassling me. At last peace and quiet and time to myself after a busy morning in the hectic house. Just watching patterns of sun and shadow dance across the outside of my tent in Pineland Park. My own world in a tall grove of trees. A snug warm cocoon. The aroma of pine needles, the sticky sap, the ocean air, and the warm sun wrap me in comfort as I lie on a bed of pine needles under the blanket rug. - **Anne**

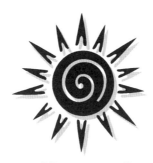

Chapter 3
Relationships: Family, Friends, and Others

"A story needs two things to live: mouths to tell it and ears to hear."
Leonard J. Pitts, Jr., *Miami Herald*, March 29, 2009

The human brain is a mysterious organ, perhaps the most complex object in the universe. When something goes wrong with it, there's no telling what the outcome might be. Since your injury, you have experienced changes in yourself. They can be physical, mental, or emotional—or all three. Some might be hardly noticeable, while others might feel overwhelming. At the same time, your family and friends might not understand how you are different, so they may be confused about how to treat you or what to expect in their relationship with you. Like you, they might be frightened or angry, or they simply might not have had time to adjust yet. The whole family is living a new story, except that no one prepared them for it or gave them a script to follow. After a brain injury of any family member, lives and relationships can be topsy-turvy for a while, like bits of paper thrown into the wind. If you are among the survivors able to find a safe, solid landing place on which to pull the pieces together again, that can take some time.

After a painful or traumatic experience, telling your story to others can be difficult. You might not yet understand what's happening. You might not be able to find the words because the changes are so large or confusing. Perhaps your brain injury prevents you from accessing the right words. You might be afraid of what others will say if you bare your soul. You might be nervous about revealing how someone's words or actions hurt you, or how you might have hurt someone. If you sense that loved ones are not yet ready to accept the new reality, that can cause you to hold back.

Fortunately, you can help your loved ones (and other people) by telling your new story through journaling with this book. Since the writing you do here is private, you can use this book first to tell your story to yourself. You can use a prompt several times, rewriting as much as you like, testing various versions to see what feels best and most true. (Each time you repeat a prompt, your entry will likely be different than previous ones, and they can all be true at the time you write them). Then, when you are comfortable with what you have written, you may choose to share your story with others to help them understand, too.

My Story 3-1
Once Upon a Time

For the first entry here, instead of using "I" to write about yourself, use "he" or "she." By writing about yourself this way—as if you were writing about someone else—you can often see a situation from a different viewpoint and learn something new. Also, using the familiar fairy tale opening "Once upon a time" can make it easier to write about something painful or difficult by creating a little distance between the event and the emotions connected with it.

```
Once upon a time, there was a person named Ken, who had a
brain injury and he was completely lost for a few weeks with no
memory of what had happened to him and how he came to feel so
very unconnected to life or even himself. After a month he was
able to talk but not connect as he still couldn't remember what
had happened even a few minutes ago. Slowly, as in much more
slowly than ever before, things began to work again. The memory
didn't work as it had, the words didn't come as easily as they
had. Many of the mental functions didn't work as they had but
they were beginning to work again. Now, 4½ years later, things
are still coming back. Going back to work has helped and being
put into a challenging area has been rough but also helped. I
don't feel as hazy as I did for so long and I'm getting better at
holding a thought long enough to see it through to a conclusion
to solve a mystery in whatever I'm doing. - Ken

Once upon a time, there was a person named Kirsten, who had
multiple "mild" brain injuries, and he/she was like the fish that
Ellen Degeneress plays in "Finding Nemo" with short-term memory
loss or what is known as anterograde amnesia—the inability to
form new memories. - Kirsten
```

☞ Choose one of these prompts:

Date: _____

✎ Once upon a time, there was a person named   (your name) , who had a brain injury, and he/she…

☞ Now, use "I." Your entry might be similar to the one above, or it might be very different. However it turns out, it is fine.

Date: _____

✎ Once upon a time, my brain was injured, and since then I…

42 After Brain Injury: Telling Your Story

My Story 3-2
Explaining My Injury

When someone breaks a leg or an arm, for example, the injury is obvious to others. However, damage to a brain may be invisible on the ouside, and so other people might misjudge or not understand the behavior of a person with a brain injury. They don't understand why you often can't find the right words to express yourself, or why you might not behave appropriately for the situation, or why you don't process or react as quickly as you did before, or why you tire easily. This means you can find yourself in the position of having to explain what it's like to live with such an injury.

```
I look normal but my thinker doesn't work so well any more.
- Ken
```

Of course, all brain injuries are as individual as the people who have sustained one, so there is no single explanation or description that will cover all brain injuries. What do you say to people when you find it necessary to explain your injury and what happened to you as a result? Do you say different things to different people? Have you created a standard explanation that you use for everyone, or does it depend on the situation?

☞ Choose one of these prompts:

Date: _____
- ✎ The major explanation I often use to tell others about my brain injury is...
- ✎ If I could tell everyone in the world this one thing about having a brain injury, I would...
- ✎ If I told ___(person's name)___ something about my injury that he or she didn't yet know, it would be...
- ✎ Freewrite...

My Story 3-3
Understanding

This prompt is good to use when it's hard for other people to understand the changes the brain injury caused in you. By writing about the changes you see in yourself or your life, you can discover more about them. And then if you want to, you can share those discoveries with others.

```
   What people don't understand about me since my brain injury is
that I'm still that intelligent, articulate, funny person and
this often masks the struggles I face daily because my executive
functions—the ability to write, summarize, create a plan,
organized, take action, self-monitor and take in corrective
feedback gracefully are things I struggle with daily. Yet, I'm
still a good person with feelings and dreams just like anyone
else. - Kirsten
```

Date: _____
- 🖋 What I don't understand about myself since my brain injury is…
- 🖋 What people don't understand about me since my brain injury is…

If you want to explain the changes to a specific person, you can use this:
- 🖋 What you don't understand about me since my brain injury is…
- 🖋 Freewrite...

My Story 3-4
Writing a Letter

One way to tell a story is to write a letter. As you know from using this workbook, telling your story doesn't require a complex plot or long words. Simply explaining why you feel the way you do can be a story, as is telling someone what happened to you today. Of course, your stories also can be much deeper and more complex than that.

The great thing about writing a letter is that you can send it—or not. Writing a letter you know you will *not* send can be an empowering, healthy way of releasing thoughts or emotions you might not feel comfortable sharing out loud or in person. You can be brutally honest. You can let 'er rip on the page, expressing anything you need to get off your chest. You can be happy or grief-stricken, calm or angry. You can tell someone how they helped you or held you back. You can simply explain how it feels to have a brain injury. You can write absolutely anything you want.

```
Hello, Mr. Brain
Please forgive me for not keeping you safe. I should of been
wearing a helmet to keep you protected. You need to know that I'm
here to protect you and try to get you back in first class shape
again. I will try to make good decisions that will keep us safe.
```
– **Michael**

```
Dear Rehab Program,
I want to tell you this about my brain injury: when coming
back into awareness, the Drs., nurses, techs & therapists that I
began to be able to see & understand during my awakening
conscious [consciousness], their compassion, caring words &
attitude match their bodies energy. The selection & hiring
process of the staff that helped make a difference in my recovery
are Susan, Jill, Jen, Kim, Kaira, & Tara. Their energies made so
much of a healing difference, better than my confussed and
frustrated families, thank you. -
```
Todd

Then, once you have written your letter, you can choose to put it away or tear it up. No one ever has to see it. On the other hand, you may want to write and send a positive letter to someone who has helped you or been especially kind.

☞ For this exercise, write a letter about your brain injury to someone who has been involved in your recovery in some way. That person can be your spouse or partner, child, other family member, friend, doctor, therapist, co-worker, or anyone else. You can even write a letter to yourself, or to your brain. Just be as honest as you can.

Then, choose one of these prompts:

Date: _____

- Dear _____,
   What I want to tell you about my brain injury is…

- Dear _____,
   Since my brain injury, I've noticed that I feel a certain way when I'm around you, and that way…

- Dear _____,
   Now that I'm working hard on my recovery from brain injury, I don't feel like you're helping me because…

- Dear _____,
   It's harder now to express myself, and it might be hard for you to understand what's happening with me, so I want to explain…

- Dear _____,
   I'd like to thank you for…

You can begin your letter any way you like, starting with:
- Dear _____,

My Story 3-5
What I Really Need

Depending on the severity of your brain injury or the changes it caused in you, your family and friends (and co-workers or fellow students, too) might have a difficult time adjusting to the changes. They might treat you differently than they used to. They don't intend to, but they may not know how to act around you or with you—and this in turn can make it difficult for you to know how to act. You can help them by writing about how you would like to be treated.

```
   Sometimes people try to help me by guessing what I want or
mean. What would really help me instead is for people to back off
and give me space and time. I'm still a person. My brain was
hurt, but I am still Elizabeth. I need some extra time. I can
answer for myself. I'm not helpless. Sometimes people treat me
like I'm dumb now. I'm not. Look at me and listen. Don't talk for
me! - Elizabeth

   Sometimes too much is going on around me and it feels like my
brain is overloaded. When this happens, I would like everyone to
stop the noise and jam in my head. It's too much! Now nothing is
working. Help bring me back to a calm place. Say things one at a
time. One person talk at a time and with one idea. Slow down.
Turn the tv off. Maybe give me and my brain a rest. Look at me.
Can't you tell it's too much now? - Oliver
```

☞ Here are some prompts you can use:

Date: _____
- Sometimes people try to help me by guessing what I want or mean. What would really help me instead is…
- Now I'm nervous when…
- Sometimes too much is going on around me and it feels like my brain is overloaded. When this happens, I would like…
- Sometimes it feels like people are looking at me differently now. What I want them to know is…
- While I can no longer do some of the things I used to do, now I can…
- Freewrite...

After Brain Injury: Telling Your Story 47

My Story 3-6
Confusing Changes

You also might feel confused about how to act with your loved ones. You might feel disappointed or angry that you can no longer do the things you used to do with them or for them. Perhaps you can no longer work, or you have to take a job that is less challenging and pays less. Perhaps your spouse has to take on more of the responsibility in the family, and you're worried about that. Perhaps your children don't understand why you can no longer coach them in sports or help with school projects. Perhaps your friends are not coming around much anymore or not asking you to join them in favorite activities you used to do together.

☞ You can write about all these things. Here are some prompts:

Date: _____
- My memory is not as good as it used to be, and …
- Just because I had a brain injury doesn't mean I can't…
- When I get upset or angry because I can no longer _____, it would help me to…
- I may not participate in the household like I used to, but what I can do now is…
- Even though we can't do _____ together anymore, we can still…
- Freewrite...

My Story 3-7
Loneliness

It's common for people with brain injury to feel lonely and isolated. Even though they may be surrounded by family and friends, they may not be able to connect with them in the same way as before the injury. New limitations on physical or mental abilities can make it more difficult to stay in touch or do favorite activities with others. Other survivors find that their family and friends are unable or unwilling to make adjustments in order to continue formerly good relationships.

```
I'm nervous around other people because I can't predict what I
might do or say. My speech therapist says my injury affected the
part of my brain that helps me monitor myself. I was in a
restaurant with my Mom last week, and I yelled at the waitress
when she brought the food. I just blurted out these words. I
don't even know what they were. From the look on her face and
Mom, I knew I had done something wrong. I didn't do it on
purpose! It just came right out of my brain through my big mouth.
I guess I do this a lot, and my friends don't want to go out with
me now. I know that Mom is getting nervous about taking me
anywhere even though she says she loves me no matter what
happens. I'm starting to feel so alone. - Michelle
```

Whatever the situation, it is important to deal in a positive way with loneliness and to find ways to maintain relationships or establish others. Please consider talking with a counselor or joining a support group for persons with brain injury to find some emotional support.

☞ Here are some prompts to use for writing about loneliness. This might be a difficult subject to write about, so if at all possible keep going for the full number of minutes you have chosen (10 to 20 minutes). By keeping your pen moving on the page or your fingers on the keyboard, your deeper thoughts can rise to the surface and come into the light. You might be surprised at how much you really know and how much you already understand. Even if the writing makes you uncomfortable at first, releasing these thoughts may soon help you feel better and stronger.

Date: _____
- ✎ I feel lonely these days because…
- ✎ Since my injury I have too many lonely "rainy days" when I look out the window and…
- ✎ People don't understand what I'm going through now and…
- ✎ My old friends don't call or invite me to join them anymore, and …
- ✎ I'm doing my best to keep my friendships going, but…
- ✎ I'm nervous around other people now because…
- ✎ It's hard for me to communicate well with people now and…
- ✎ I still love my spouse/partner very much, but it's more difficult now to show that because…
- ✎ Since my brain injury, my spouse/partner doesn't seem to want to…
- ✎ I'm afraid I'll never find a good relationship now because…
- ✎ Freewrite…

After Brain Injury: Telling Your Story

My Story 3-8
Overcoming Loneliness

You can take action to reduce and overcome your loneliness. Remember that both people in a relationship have something to offer, and they must both contribute to the relationship and work to the best of their abilities to keep it healthy.

A few ways you can contribute to your relationships:

- ✓ Do your best to be a friendly, welcoming person.
- ✓ Develop activities you enjoy doing on your own. This will make you a more interesting companion and give you something to talk about.
- ✓ Look for the positive qualities in yourself and others.

```
The people in my life who can help me when I need help are
mostly women.  There are a few men that will respond but for me I
find it is women's hearts that make the difference in my feeling
safe.  There are the funny ones that make me laugh!  The wise
ones, that become my Mentors. The quiet ones that listen deeply
and let me cry. The movers and shakers, that give me courage to
be me. - Lela
```

☞ Write about some actions you can take to overcome loneliness and improve relationships with these prompts:

Date: _____
- ✎ Something I can do to improve my relationships is…
- ✎ Even though my relationships have changed, I can still show people I care for them by…
- ✎ It's more difficult now to have a good time with my family and friends, but I can still…
- ✎ I can help my family and friends feel more comfortable with me by…
- ✎ I can be a good friend by…
- ✎ Someone I would like to resume a relationship with…
- ✎ I can make an effort to make new friends by…
- ✎ A new relationship I developed recently…

☞ Your family members and friends might want to remain close with you, but they may not know or understand what you need and want in a relationship now. You can write about how they can help you with this. If you like, you can then show them what you have written. Here are some prompts for this:

- ✎ I know that our relationship has changed since my brain injury, and something you could do to help me is…
- ✎ It's harder now for me to understand what other people are thinking and feeling, so when we're together, you could help me by…
- ✎ When we're doing something together, I would feel more comfortable if you would…
- ✎ I appreciate that you're being so helpful to me now because…
- ✎ Freewrite...

My Story 3-9
Asking for Help, Part 1

Probably one of the hardest things for adults to do is give up their independence. When they don't have to depend on others too much, it's a sign that they can take care of themselves, that they're doing fine. The so-called American tradition of independence only adds to those feelings.

But here's a secret: None of us is truly independent in the sense that we never need help from anyone else. Every day, everyone needs assistance with the tasks of living!

Consider this: Even before your brain injury, would you have been able to find enough food, clothe yourself, or have work and money if you never received help from anyone? Can you imagine a household or a city or a country where no one helped anyone else? If you never requested or received help, you wouldn't live very long. That is why everything on the planet is *inter*dependent. You depend on others for some things and they depend on you for some things. All the pieces fit together in a huge, complex web that forms the whole. So, while you can be independent in some areas, you are much more interconnected in many other ways.

In fact, true independence deals much more with how you feel inside than with what is happening to you on the outside. Even if your injury means you now need more assistance with activities of daily living, you can still maintain a strong inner sense of independence. First of all, accepting that you legitimately need help with certain things will hold down your stress and frustration levels. Some people require a cane or walker in order to walk safely; refusing to use this kind of helpful tool makes no sense and only limits them. For you to refuse legitimate assistance when you truly need it will limit you as well. Furthermore, graciously asking for and accepting help when necessary allows you to maintain your sense of self-identity as well as your dignity (and also provides dignity to your helper). At the same time, you should also feel free to politely refuse help when you don't need it.

You probably still want to do all the things you used to do, and do them equally well if at all possible. That's normal, commendable, and totally understandable. Yet challenges arise when the injury prevents you from going to work or school, driving, reading, playing with your children, taking a walk, cooking, learning, remembering, cleaning the house, tying your shoes, using the television remote, using your computer, or any number of things. Even if your ability to do these things is only reduced or diminished, that can still be frustrating.

Let's face it—as an adult, it can be embarrassing to have to ask for help with something you've been able to do for years, maybe even since childhood. On top of that, you might be afraid that people, even your nearest and dearest, will give up on you if you ask for help too many times. You might find yourself wondering, "If they don't want to help me, how will I manage?"

First of all, know that many resources are available. There is a short list in the back of this workbook, and you can find many more on the Internet or your local library. Additionally, you can journal about your frustrations with having to ask for help *and* about your successes and achievements.

☞ Here are some prompts you can start with:

Date: _____
This prompt has two parts.

First part:
- Before my brain injury, asking for help…

Second part:
- Now that I need help more often, I…

☞ Additional prompts:

Date: _____
- I hate having to ask for help because…
- It's OK for me to ask for help because…
- Now that I have to rely more on other people…
- It's getting easier to do things on my own and…
- I feel proud of myself for asking for help because…
- I used to need help with…
- Freewrite…

My Story 3-10
Asking for Help, Part 2

Being embarrassed may cause you to lash out at people, even if they were being helpful. When someone volunteers to help you with a task, how do you treat that person? What about when someone assumes you need help you don't actually need—are you polite and thankful when you refuse their assistance or do you snarl?

When you ask for help, do people agree easily or happily? Or do they show their displeasure? How do you feel then?

Realize that you and your helpers are both part of the "helping equation." Although you cannot be responsible for how the other person feels or acts, you can often gain more control over yourself.

☞ So, without denying your feelings and by writing honestly about being helped, you may understand yourself better and so improve the situation. Try these prompts:

Date: _____
- Having to ask for your help so often embarrasses me, and…
- I know I haven't always been pleasant when asking for your help, so…
- Thank you for helping me with _____ because…
- I'm so happy you're here to help me because…
- A time I asked for help and got a negative reaction was…
- A time I asked for help and got a postive reaction was…
- Freewrite...

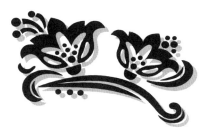

Chapter 4
Adjustments: Anger and Grief

"In a dark time, the eye begins to see."
Theodore Roethke, "In a Dark Time"

A brain injury is a frightening, life-altering event. The ultimate outcome, dependent on so many circumstances and details, can never be predicted. Yet because an injury to the brain often rips away portions of an identity and alters the direction of a familiar life, survivors need to find a way to deal in a healthy manner with their grief and anger at these unexpected changes. Then eventually they may discover hope and rebuild their lives, sometimes along a wildly new path. It's important to remember that even though such a life may be much different than life before the injury, it can still be heartfelt, satisfying, and productive.

One important key to creating your new life is telling the story of your anger and grief. Write about them as often as necessary, with all the honesty and freedom available to you, and watch your progress over time. By communicating with your inner self in this way and giving it a voice on paper, you are choosing to move forward.

However, when you let anger overwhelm you so that you cannot rationally or calmly deal with a situation, it can be harmful. At the least, it prevents you from exploring other options to the problem; at the worst, it can push you into hurting yourself or someone else. Remember, it is always helpful to work with a trusted person, such as a counselor or therapist, who can guide you through your dark times and emotions.

My Story 4-1
Telling the Story of My Anger

Anger is a common reaction to unexpected events that do harm and throw you off-course. It's a way of coping emotionally with the situation until you can either make sense of it or make peace with it. After a brain injury, you could be angry at yourself— "Why did I ride my bike without a helmet, just that one time?" You could be angry at the person who caused the injury— "That idiot swung the bat and didn't look to see if anyone was behind him!" Sometimes you might be angry at the circumstances even though there was nothing you could have done about them— "I was serving in the military in Iraq, and that damn roadside bomb exploded just as we were driving by. Why did I enlist?" Or, "Why did I get a brain tumor? I've always taken good care of my health. This shouldn't have happened to me."

```
   I'm mad at that brown dog because if it hadn't run in front of
me, I wouldn't have swerved on my bike causing this accident.
That dog didn't know how my life would change. It probably just
kept running and is still probably running. But look at me now.
That darn dog. I don't like dogs anymore. - Carly
```

☞ Here are just a few prompts about anger. If it's difficult to give yourself permission to write about your anger, begin with the first prompt.

Date: _____

✎ If I could tell the story about what most angers me about my brain injury, I would say…

☞ Then continue with these.

✎ Something that makes me mad about my brain injury is… (You can use this as many times and for as many items as necessary.)
✎ I'm mad at myself because…
✎ It is so unfair that I have this brain injury because…
✎ I'm mad at _____ because…
✎ I get angry because no one seems to understand what I'm going through and…
✎ I know it's not my fault that I have a brain injury, but I'm angry anyway because…
✎ I know it's no one's fault that I have a brain injury, yet…
✎ I have a right to feel angry about what's happened to me …
✎ I don't want to feel angry about my brain injury, but I do because…
✎ I'm angry at God…
✎ Freewrite...

My Story 4-2
Feeling the Anger

However justified you feel in remaining angry, at some point you'll need to ask yourself what good that does. Hanging on to your anger can slow down your recovery and push away people who want to help. Consider working with a counselor or therapist experienced in brain injury if you have a hard time letting go of your anger over time, especially if you lash out at yourself or others with anger you cannot seem to control. You can also try this next exercise any time you want to let go of anger when it flares up.

```
Now I know the real source of my anger is me. I just keep
thinking about the accident over and over and over. I don't
remember much of it, but I've seen the pictures of the car, and I
just keep thinking about it. Then my head starts pounding and I
want to scream—and sometimes I do. I know I need to stop
replaying this over and over. Sometimes I think about going to
the lake and swimming when I was a little girl or running on the
beach barefooted. That calms me. My head doesn't feel like it's
going to explode. - Jillian
```

You experience your emotions in your body, even if you don't realize this as it's happening. That means you can often change the emotion by changing the physical feeling, and you can do this on purpose. Try to feel sad while smiling, for instance. If the smile is genuine, you can't feel the emotion of sadness. Try to feel peaceful while tensing your whole body. That doesn't work, either.

☞ One way to reduce anger is to pay attention to how it feels physically, and then release that physical sensation and replace it with a calmer one. So, when you wrote from the earlier prompts in "Telling the Story of My Anger," My Story 4-1, Chapter 4, ask yourself how your body experienced the anger. Did your stomach hurt or feel tied in knots? Did your heart rate speed up and your breath become shallow? Did you feel a headache coming on from tensing your neck muscles? And so on. Write about this physical feeling. It's possible you may learn more about the source of your anger.

Date: _____
- As I wrote about my anger, my body…
- While writing about being angry over my brain injury, my   (part of body)   felt as if…
- I understand now how anger makes me feel physically, and…
- Now I know the real source of my anger is…
- Freewrite…

☞ Now do this. Put down your pen or pencil and sit quietly with eyes closed, as you do for the relaxation technique. In your body, experience how it felt to be angry while writing, and then begin to take slow, deep breaths as you consciously relax your body from head to toe—your head, neck, torso, arms, hands, stomach, back, hips, legs, and feet. Keep breathing slowly and let your anger flow out of your fingertips and toes, like raindrops running down a hillside. If anger rises again, consciously relax the part of your body where you feel it, and let it flow out and away. Keep going until you can sense no remaining trace of anger or tension.

> I will replace my anger with all the good things I can do. It's a waste of energy for me to think about the surgery over and over. It happened. I'm mad, but you know, I'm still here and each day I seem to get stronger and stronger. Rehab is going well. I'm not as tired or dizzy as I used to be. I talked to my neighbor today. I haven't done that in a long time. Tomorrow I'm going to help her plant flowers—at least talk with her while she's planting them. Then she said she would show me her paintings. Who knows, maybe I can paint. It will be a challenge with my arm and eyes not working like they used to, but I'm going to give it a try. – **Josh**

☞ Now, pick up your pen or pencil again and write from one of these prompts:

Date: _____
- As I let the physical feeling of anger flow out of my body, I felt…
- In the future, when I feel my body tense with anger and I don't want to be angry, I will…
- I am willing to let go of this physical feeling of anger, and so I …
- I really wanted to release my anger, but I couldn't because…
- I am willing to replace my anger with…
- I am willing to channel my anger in a more positive direction by…
- Freewrite...

My Story 4-3
Grieving the Losses

Along with the anger you experienced after your brain injury, you likely also felt—or still feel—intense sadness, fear, regret, and hopelessness. All of these feelings are normal responses to a significant loss, and they are all part of the process of grieving. Grief is a deep sorrow we most often associate with the death of a loved one, yet it can appear anytime we lose something important to our well-being and happiness. Certainly a brain injury can lead to great losses.

```
    I feel so sad about losing my brain. Well, I didn't lose it
really but parts of it sure are gone. I can hardly write any
more, and it's hard to read now too. I used to read all the time.
It was my favorite thing to do. That means I can't go back to
school and who knows what kind of job I'll ever have. My
therapists tell me I'm making progress, be patient, keep up the
good work. But it's all so hard. It's taking so long. That driver
was drunk, and I lost so much because of him. I just want to sit
here where it's quiet and not have to talk or think. I can barely
even think without my head hurting anyway. I don't know what to
do with all this sadness I feel inside me. It hurts, even when
I'm asleep. It hurts in my dreams. Will I ever feel better? -
```
Carole, as told to Yvonne

Many survivors of brain injury have to face the realization that they may never be the same as they once were, and so they feel an intense loss of self and must mourn "the old me." Such a huge loss is a kind of emotional death, and mourning is appropriate. In fact, grief is an important part of the emotional healing process. It lets people come to terms with the new reality and clears the way for the personal growth and understanding they can use to move on with their lives.

```
    Sometimes people tell me to "snap out of it," and that makes
me so MAD. Are you my brain? Do you know what I'm going through?
Do you think I'm doing this on purpose? Try being in my head for
a day. - Allison
```

Everyone grieves in their own way and in their own time, and it is helpful for people with a brain injury to work through their grief with a counselor who understands the unique specifics of grieving after a brain injury. This workbook can cover only a few of those aspects, so here are some prompts you can use in the process. Remember that writing about your grief, even for short periods of time, may assist you in your recovery process.

☞ Just as you learned what anger felt like in your body, you can do the same with your grief. As you write about your grief, pay attention to how your body feels.

Date: _____
✎ My grief feels worst when…

- ✐ This deep sadness surrounding me…
- ✐ My grief is like…
- ✐ I feel so sad about losing…
- ✐ Because I don't know what to do with all this sadness and emotional pain, I…
- ✐ Another time I grieved about _____, and that was the same as now because…
- ✐ Another time I grieved about _____, and that was different than now because…
- ✐ Sometimes people tell me to "snap out of it," and that makes me…
- ✐ Freewrite...

Date: _____

- ✐ In your journal, make a list that begins: My grief is a jumble of so many feelings, including... (write in as many as you can discover)

☞ You can also write a letter to your grief to explain how you feel about it. Or you can dialogue with it, as you have written other dialogues in this workbook, to find out what it "says" to you. (For a reminder about writing dialogue, see My Story 1-5, Chapter 1.)

Begin with one of these:

Date: _____
- ✐ Letter to Grief
    Dear Grief,

Date: _____
- ✐ Dialogue with Grief

    Me:

    Grief:

My Story 4-4
Feeling the Grief

As you wrote about your grief, how did it feel in your body? Did the sadness turn to tears? Did your chest feel heavy, as if your heart would break? Did it feel like a weight pushing down on your shoulders?

```
   As I wrote about my grief, my body felt like it was covered by
a pile of stones, squeezing me so tight I could hardly breathe.
It was hard to move my hand to write in my journal. They are so
heavy, I can't push them off. They are going to crush me flat.
Maybe I don't care. I cry all the time. - Sam
```

☞ Write about this physical feeling of grief to understand and, if you're ready, help release it.

Date: _____
- 🖋 As I wrote about my grief, my body…
- 🖋 While writing about grieving the losses due to my brain injury, my _(part of body)_ felt as if…
- 🖋 Freewrite…

My Story 4-5
Comfort

While grieving, you need to take good care of yourself. Grieving is hard, and it hurts, but that doesn't mean you shouldn't seek out comfort. In fact, you need some healthy comforts (NOT alcohol or overeating, or drugs unless prescribed by your doctor) to help you through this time. Some examples of healthy ways to comfort yourself: read from a favorite book, watch a cheerful movie, care for your pets or even a plant, try gentle exercise if you are physically able, spend time outside, listen to uplifting music, sip hot chocolate or tea while wrapped in a comfy blanket, soak in a warm bath, or share your feelings with your journal. These comforts are small, but they are important.

☞ Do something healthy to comfort yourself as often as necessary.

Date: _____

- In your journal, make a list that begins: To comfort myself in this time of grief, I will do these positive things for myself: (See if you can write at least 5.)

- When I can, I put aside my grief, even for a few minutes, and…
- It's okay to give myself permission to find healthy comfort during this time because…
- I respect the difficult time I'm going through right now, and know that comforting myself is part of the process, so I…
- Freewrite...

My Story 4-6
Awareness, Acceptance, Acknowledgement, and Accommodation

Many people with brain injury may not return to the way they were before their injury. Their lives may be changed in some ways, perhaps drastically. Initially, their awareness of their limitations may be shallow or limited. Over time, it usually emerges and grows. (For some individuals, improvement in self-awareness is limited by damage to specific parts of the brain.) This awareness is an important step to accepting and acknowledging what has happened and how they view themselves. It is harder for them to accept help if they are not aware of their limitations or problems. As awareness continues to improve, survivors are more able to self-monitor their actions and behaviors.

```
Some of the changes I am aware of after the brain injury are
really not much. I'm feeling pretty good. I get tired quicker,
but who wouldn't? People need to stop babying me. I've driven
before—my family says I can't drive but I think I'm fine to drive
now. I'll be careful. I'll be fine. - Hilda (shallow awareness)
```

Many survivors don't want to accept what has happened because they believe acceptance means giving up hope of further recovery. They think that if they accept where they are today, they will never again move forward.

However, acceptance does *not* mean giving up. Not in the least. Accepting what has happened simply means that you realize your situation is now different than it used to be. You sustained a brain injury, and you have changed as a result. If you stubbornly refuse to accept what happened, you drain your energy by fighting against something that cannot be changed. That leaves you with little or no energy to continue making progress in your recovery.

Consider a car with a tank full of gas. If the front of the car is up against an unbreakable, unmovable wall but you refuse to accept that fact, you can start up the car and jam down the accelerator as long and as hard as you want, but you won't go anywhere. The tires will spin uselessly, mechanical parts of the car will burn out, and eventually all the gas will be used up. On the other hand, if you accept the presence of the wall, you can back up the car and then turn the wheels so you can drive in various directions. In accommodating yourself to the presence of the wall, you can move. You might have to maneuver around other obstacles, or discover that the car doesn't get the gas mileage you would like, and perhaps the radio doesn't work so well any more, but you can make progress in new directions.

```
A change I am aware of after the brain injury is that maybe
that my memory isn't as good as it used to be. My therapist wants
me to use a daily planner. I guess I missed our appointment
yesterday. I thought it was tomorrow. I don't think my memory is
that different, but Mom says I ask her the same questions again
and again. So do my friends. Maybe I just need some rest. - Lucas
(emerging awareness)
```

After Brain Injury: Telling Your Story 63

> Some of the changes I am aware of after the brain injury are that my memory and attention need work, but I'm getting there. I got a daily planner. It goes everywhere with me. I haven't missed one appointment this past week. Also, I can tell you what else I've been doing the past week. I know the score of the basketball game. I don't want to use the planner. I don't like it. But, it's better than getting yelled at by my therapist and having to ask others to repeat everything. I feel I'm more on my own that way. I have also learned I need to do one thing at a time now. No TV while I'm talking to someone. A list and shopping early in the morning. I have one place now for my glasses—haven't lost them the past week. Same thing with my cell phone. Getting back on track. – **Roy** (self-monitoring)

☞ Here are some prompts about becoming aware of your post-injury changes, accepting and acknowledging them, and then accommodating them to find new directions. You can use these many times as your awareness emerges and evolves over time.

Awareness
Date: _____
- Some of the changes I became aware of after the brain injury are…
- After my brain injury, I remember becoming aware of changes in me or in my life when…
- This awareness felt…
- I'd rather not have this awareness because…
- I'm happy to have this awareness because…
- My awareness is growing, and…
- My awareness of my situation is…
- I'm aware that my brain injury will affect my family and friends by…
- I'm aware that my brain injury will affect my job by…
- I'm aware that my brain injury will affect my schooling by…
- Freewrite…

Acceptance and Acknowledgment
Date: _____
- I still have not been able to accept the changes due to my brain injury because…
- I don't want to accept the changes that occurred after my brain injury…
- Maybe I can begin to accept some of the changes if…
- Instead of using the word "accept" when talking about how I'm adjusting to the changes due to my brain injury, I prefer to use the word _____ because…
- I was finally able to accept the changes caused by my brain injury when…
- I now accept that my life…
- I now accept that I…
- Freewrite…

Accommodation
People with a paralyzing spinal cord injury use wheelchairs in order to be mobile. Near-sighted people use glasses or contact lenses to see clearly. In the same way, people with brain injury can use various devices and strategies to accommodate some losses and enhance their remaining strengths. For instance, survivors with certain memory problems can use special calendars or devices to keep track of

daily events. Other survivors may be able to use cell phones to play videos that lead them through certain tasks, such as brushing their teeth. If survivors can no longer drive, they may be able to use public transportation. Special eyeglasses called prism glasses allow survivors with certain optic disabilities to expand their visual field. Many more accommodations can be devised with the help of therapists and other professionals with experience in brain injury.

What kind of accommodations have you made to allow yourself to live a more fulfilling life? Are you resisting certain accommodations? Are you excited to find new ways of adapting to your new situation?

☞ Write from these prompts to explore these issues:

Date: _____
- I can't do _____ any longer, but instead I can…
- Some strategies I've learned for enhancing my strengths are…
- It's very hard to adjust to…
- Even though I understand why it might be necessary for me to use certain accommodations for my brain injury, I'm still resisting because…
- Instead of wasting my energy with _____, I choose to use my energy in a positive way by…
- At first after my injury, I refused to use _____, but now I use it because…
- It's exciting to find new methods that allow me to…
- In order to move ahead in my recovery, I choose to adapt to…
- Freewrite...

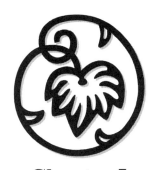

Chapter 5
Back Into the Community: Moving Forward With Hope

"Our responsibility, then, is to find and know the story that is our own."
Gertrud Mueller Nelson, *All Dwell Free*

"I am the only one who can tell the story of my life and say what it means."
Dorothy Allison, *Bastard Out of Carolina*

This section will allow you to explore your feelings about going back into the world after your brain injury rehabilitation. Your therapists and doctors probably have called this "community re-entry." It is a time of moving forward. It might mean leaving the protected environment of a rehabilitation center to experience daily life outside its walls. This life will be full of those activities that people normally do in our society—some of which you may not be able to do now, or not as well as before.

If your brain injury happened some time ago and you have already made your re-entry into the community, don't skip this section. There are many prompts here, and some of them might appeal to you as well.

A major part of community re-entry and moving forward is seeking out the hope that exists in your situation, and learning how to stay as hopeful and positive as possible. There will be prompts related to hope later in this section, but first, you can make your declaration of what your life means to you.

My Story 5-1
What Your Life Means

Just as Dorothy Allison proclaims in the quote above, the only person who can say what your life means is *you*. Even if you have a brain injury, you must tell your own story to decide what your life means. If you don't, how will you be able to figure out what you want your life to be now? And how else will other people understand who you are and how you want to lead your life?

```
    To be able to live my life on my own terms, I need to be clear
in my own mind, and to others, by what I allow or say. If I don't
set limits it's way too easy to become overwhelmed. I'm the only
one who knows what I can do and how I need to do it. My new
limits only allow so much leeway as how I approach a task at work
and at home. It takes me longer, sometimes several tries, to get
a task or conversation known enough in my mind to be able to move
forward. If I don't "get it" immediately, it doesn't mean I
didn't hear. It may well mean I must mull it over a number of
times before it becomes clear to me. I know I'm not stupid, just
running fewer than "all cylinders" these days. I must become
demanding so to give myself the best chance to still be valuable
at home and at work. - Ken
```

Sometimes, others will define you by what they think you have lost. And they also may expand a single loss into further deficits. Have you ever seen someone talking loudly to a blind person, as if being unable to see means loss of hearing? It's a misplaced impulse caused by ignorance (even if the intention is positive). Fortunately, you can educate people about your life after a brain injury by telling your stories. Like the bricks that make up a building, you use small stories to create a larger whole, the new Story of Your Life.

☞ Even if the brain injury has made you more dependent on others than you used to be, or if you cannot do some of the things you used to do, you are still allowed to determine the meaning of your life to the extent your abilities permit. Try these prompts on this subject:

Date: _____
✎ To be able to live my life on my own terms, I need…
✎ I am the only one who can say what my life means, and I say it means…
✎ I want to lead my life in a way that…
✎ My own story of going back out in the world is telling me…
✎ Freewrite...

My Story 5-2
Hope in Your Future

Every brain injury is unique. Recovery depends on many elements, including the severity and location of the injury, medical and rehabilitation care, quality of the support system, the person's determination and motivation, and activities and education levels before the injury. Not too many years ago, the standard belief was that recovery, if any, would occur up to the two-year mark; after that, there was not much hope for more progress. Fortunately, new research has shown that healing and further recovery from brain injury can continue for many years, perhaps for a lifetime. There is always hope, if not for full recovery, than perhaps for much more recovery than was believed possible in the past. Many survivors have a great deal of inner drive and personal strength they can call upon to re-make their lives—if they have hope. (There are many good books written by or about people with brain injury who sought and sustained their hope. Please see the list of resources at the back of this book.)

Do you feel hopeful regarding your future? Do you believe your life can be satisfying and productive after your brain injury, even if it might be much different than it used to be? There is an old saying, "Where there is life, there is hope." Do you believe it? Even if you do most of the time, it's likely that your level of hope will vary from day to day. You will probably go through periods when you feel ambivalent about your new self. At times, you may believe the brain injury gave you a second chance, and other times, it will feel like a gigantic burden. On those days when your hope levels are low or you are confused about how you feel, give yourself permission to admit that and write about it. You may find that rays of hope and clarity will emerge in your writing. Even with the difficulties in your life, you may still find resilience, wisdom, and courage within yourself.

```
One thing that gives me hope after my TBI [traumatic brain
injury] happened at work within a few weeks of my return a full 6
months since the TBI. I'd been warned that suicide is common post
TBI and I was starting to think about suicide as my feelings of
hopelessness increased. I was at work only two hours a day then
as I couldn't handle any more. I went out for a walk thinking
about what it would take to be willing to commit suicide. First I
would have to know what I had been pre TBI. Second I would have
to know what I was post TBI. Thirdly I would have to be able to
hold both thoughts so I could compare them. I could do all three
of those thoughts and it made me very despondent to know the
difference between the was-me and the is-me. I also knew there
would have to be another part to all this that would push me over
the edge. The other piece would be lack of hope. What makes hope?
Seeing improvement brings hope. For me cognitive thought is hope.
I walked slowly and thought more about all this in my then
pondering fashion. Then I really got it. Handling what was, what
is, and making a comparison between the two major items is a
cognitive thought! What I needed most was in front of me all the
time. Knowing I could still think gave me hope and the intention
to continue healing. All thoughts of suicide left and haven't
been back. I still have up and down days but I always know I'm
still here to keep going and healing for as long as I can. - Ken
```

☞ Choose from these prompts based on how you feel at the time of writing:

Date: _____
- One thing that gives me the most hope after my brain injury is…
- I have hope for continued recovery because I see small bits of progress happening, and they are…
- Even after brain injury, I see a hopeful bridge to my future, and it…
- Even with a brain injury, I have a second chance at life, and…
- Something hopeful that happened in the past week…
- Sometimes I feel hopeless about my recovery because…
- Even though I don't feel very hopeful today, I know I will later because…
- Two people who influence my hope are…
- Two events or things that influence my hope are…
- Freewrite…

My Story 5-3
Nurturing Hope

Sometimes when you're having a bad day—or a lousy week or terrible month—you have to actively nurture hope and other positive feelings within yourself, just as a gardener tends a delicate plant to keep it alive and thriving. During these difficult times, you must be kind to yourself, and you must also encourage yourself. The word "encourage" comes from two words that together mean to "make or put in courage," and the word "courage" comes from an Old French word meaning "heart," as it refers to feelings. So, to encourage yourself means to put your heart-feelings into whatever task you are doing. When it comes to maintaining hope, then, you must look deep in your heart to find the feelings and thoughts that will keep you hope-full. Even when you can find only the tiniest seed of hope, it will grow if you cherish and nurture it.

☞ Here are some prompts about hope:

Date: _____
- I encourage myself to remain hopeful by…
- I applaud myself for the efforts I am making to recover as much as possible, even when…
- It takes a lot of courage to live with a brain injury, and I maintain my courage by…
- When I lose hope, the world around me looks like…
- When I'm full of hope, the world around me looks like…
- I'm more able to be kind and gentle with myself when I feel hopeful because…
- Freewrite…

My Story 5-4
Asking Others to Hope With You

When the people around you don't encourage your feelings of hope, you can lose heart. However, you can write about why having hope is so important to you, and then you can share your writing with others. That way you can encourage them to encourage you!

```
    Thank you so much for being hopeful for me, Dad. I know that
you won't leave me or look at me like I'm stupid or crazy when I
can't talk right or lose my balance. You know I'm not crazy or
stupid you know I'm working hard as I can to get better from my
accident. Mom is sad around me all the time now, and that makes
me even sadder, but you still laugh with me. You cheer me up. You
rented that old Marx Brothers movie, the one where all those
people pile into a little room and then someone opens the door
and they all fall out. You were laughing so hard! And I thought I
would never stop laughing. Thanks, Dad. You make me feel like I'm
still a real person.
    Love, Sam, your son - Sam
```

☞ Write about what hope means to you and why it is important.

Date:_____
- It's important for me to stay hopeful about recovering as much as I can, so I would appreciate it if you would help me by…
- I'm encouraging myself to remain hopeful about my recovery, and you will encourage me, too, if you would…
- Thank you so much for being hopeful about my recovery and future life because…
- I appreciate that you're helping me to remain hopeful by…
- When I am not hopeful, please…
- Freewrite...

My Story 5-5
Your Home

After your brain injury, you may have spent time in a hospital and possibly a rehabilitation center, both of which are protected environments. Then you were released to go home. Whether you live alone or with other people, the place where you live now is not as protected or structured as the rehab center, so you must begin dealing with "life on the outside" again. That alone can be stressful, but on top of that, your home might feel different to you now. Perhaps memory loss has made it feel less familiar, or perhaps it's just plain uncomfortable for some reason. Maybe your home requires changes to accommodate you now, like a wheelchair ramp to the front door or grab bars in the bathtub. Or you might have to accommodate yourself to the house because physical changes are not possible.

```
Being back home was a big event for me. I had not seen my home
for four months. I was nervous in the car with Tom when we left
the rehab center. I wondered how I would feel back in my own bed.
Would I still be able to go out in the back to work on my roses?
I hadn't cooked for four months either, and I used to be such a
good cook. Everyone said so. I know I made an omlet in rehab. It
was a test and Tom and I ate the omelet for lunch. He looked so
proud. When we got home the neighbors were waiting with flowers
and big smiles and balloons. The house felt huge inside. I felt
so overwhelmed. - Pat
```

In the 2001 movie *Life As a House*, the main character says, "I always thought of myself as a house. I was always what I lived in. It didn't need to be big. It didn't even need to be beautiful. It just needed to be mine. I became what I was meant to be. I built myself a life. I built myself a house." After a brain injury, you may need to redefine what you were "meant to be" as you build a new life, including perhaps the part of your life you experience within the walls of your home.

It can be enlightening to explore your home, to see how you feel about it now—be it a house, an apartment, a mobile home, an RV, even an assisted living arrangement. With journaling, you can discover how you feel—physically, emotionally, spiritually, and mentally—about being home, which in turn can reveal insights about other parts of your life. Go through your home and use your senses to explore the rooms—what do you see, smell, touch, feel, hear, or taste? If you like, draw a map of your home in your journal and in each of the rooms write the words that describe what your senses tell you there.

☞ Next, do the relaxation technique on page 10, and then begin to write. Explore whatever feelings come.

Date: _____
- If I were this house, I…
- I am a house, and…
- Being back home…
- This place where I live now feels…
- It's hard to live here now because…
- It's comforting to live here now because…
- When I explore this place where I live, I find…
- Freewrite...

My Story 5-6
A Letter from Home

It can be enlightening to see yourself from another's perspective—especially if you use your imagination to create that perspective. What if your home wrote a letter to you, explaining how it feels about having you back, or how it sees you now?

Just as you wrote a letter to someone or something in other sections of this workbook, you can imagine yourself to be your home and write a letter to you. What would your home want you to know now? Does it have some news or questions to share with you? Perhaps your home simply wants to "talk" with you, its old friend, to renew your acquaintance and get settled into the new life you will both share. If you're living in a new place, it can introduce itself.

☞ In this letter, imagine that you are this structure that shelters you, and see what this letter from Home says.

Date: _____

- Dear ___(your name)___,
  Now that you're back within my walls, I feel…

- Dear ___(your name)___,
  I'm so glad you're back! While you were gone…

- Dear ___(your name)___,
  This isn't a good place for you to be…

- Dear ___(your name)___,
  This is a good place for you to be…

- Dear ___(your name)___,
  (begin writing in your own words)

74 After Brain Injury: Telling Your Story

My Story 5-7
New People

Some of the changes you have undergone may not be noticeable to others, even though they feel huge to you. Other changes might be very apparent to other people but not to you. Is there a difference in what you notice about yourself and what others notice? Does it make you uncomfortable for others to notice, or not? How do you deal with feeling uncomfortable around new people?

```
Since my injury, the thing I notice most within myself is that
I'm my most harsh critic and that my demands of myself need to be
softened and that I need to learn to treat myself with kindness
and gentleness, as would say a child who was struggling to manage
a barrage of emotions/feelings and didn't know how. I need to
have patience with myself that I would naturally give a small
child.
    The thing other people notice most about me is that it is hard
for me to be real with some people because so much of my current
life is spent dealing daily with physical health crises, systems
crises, and emotional health melt downs. That I'm in a state of
perpetual chronic stress and I'm so tired cognitively and I have
very little patience with myself (this aptly describes my
unsupportive family, too). The people who support me notice how
many new skills I'm slowly acquiring as habits and see me making
more good choices than bad. There are still times when they might
not be happy with how I behave and this doesn't mean they stay
mad at me. They just want to see some of the major traumas in my
life healed and that is happening slowly. - Kirsten

    People simply don't get it. I mean I look pretty good. If I
mention my memory sometimes not working as well or that I can't
find my words like I used to, people will often gloss over the
situation with a response such as I know what you mean or who
says getting older was easy? People simply don't get it! - Randy
```

When you begin venturing out into the world again, you will come across many people you don't know. They won't know about your injury or the challenges you face. They might be rude or treat you unkindly, or they might as easily be pleasant and helpful. How do you deal with these situations? Remember that each situation is unique, and you can write about various situations as they occur. If you see that you react in ways you're not happy about, you can imagine better ways to act and write about that. You may remember it for the next time.

> ☞ Writing with these prompts can help you discover how to handle situations in which you or others feel uncomfortable. It can change or improve how you feel about yourself or help you develop a positive strategy for dealing with these feelings. You also might realize you don't mind being "different" than you used to be or that you're comfortable with your new self, regardless of what others may think. You may find interactions to be better than before.

Date: _____
- ✎ Since my injury, the change I notice most about myself is…
- ✎ Since my injury, the change I think other people notice most about me is...
- ✎ When I see that other people think I'm different, I feel…
- ✎ When strangers are rude or unkind to me, I…
- ✎ If I need help when I'm out by myself, I tell people I have a brain injury because…
- ✎ If I need help when I'm out by myself, I do not tell people I have a brain injury because…
- ✎ When I'm with people who don't know me, I'm afraid I might…
- ✎ When I've been around strangers, I have done things I don't feel good about, and those things are…
- ✎ When I'm with strangers, I feel confident I can…
- ✎ I'm not pleased with how I reacted to __(describe event)__ and so next time, I will…
- ✎ Freewrite...

My Story 5-8
Making Your Way Around

At some point in your recovery, you will begin making your way into the community again. At first you may need assistance or someone to guide you. Eventually you'll probably begin going out on your own. No matter how easy it was for you to navigate around your city or town before your injury, now you might find it difficult. You might be frightened about getting lost when the surroundings don't look familiar or because your navigating skills or memory have been affected. A speech or occupational therapist can help you with strategies for making your way around your community.

☞ Unless you plan to never leave your house again, you will be living a new story out in the world, too. Writing about it over time will let you record your progress (and your adventures!). Here are some prompts:

Date: _____
- When I go out by myself now, I am…
- When I leave the house on my own now, the city or town where I live feels…
- It's difficult to leave the house on my own because…
- I feel brave enough to go out alone because…
- I can hardly wait to go out alone because…
- I look fine, so people…
- I really want to go __(place)__ because…
- Now that I'm able to go out on my own, I can look forward to…
- I went out alone today and…
- I went by myself to __(place)__, and what happened was…
- If I go out alone and get lost, I will…
- In order to not get lost, I will…
- Freewrite...

My Story 5-9
Work Issues

Most adults define themselves in large part through their work. The world tends to use that same definition: when people meet for the first time a typical question is, "What do you do?" Whether it takes place in an office, factory, store, or other setting, work is where most adults spend a third (or more) of their lives, feel productive, make friends, and connect with the larger community. And, just like those who work outside the home, stay-at-home parents gain satisfaction from their work—the essential role of caring for their homes and families.

When someone of working age is not employed, it's common to feel isolated and left out. When stay-at-home parents can no longer fill the same household roles as before, they may feel adrift or useless. Adding a brain injury into the mix, with the uncertainty of being able to return to the same job or sometimes to any work at all, only increases the stress and uneasiness.

Other issues also arise. If the survivor of a brain injury is unable to bring home the same level of pay, the spouse may have to make up for the missing income. This can cause stress for the couple, and for the entire family. Having to take a less-demanding job or one with a "lower" status, even temporarily, may feel embarrassing or demeaning, and may be resisted. Some survivors might feel the same way about having to go on disability, whether it's short-term or permanent. While some are excited about going back to work, others might not be able to overcome their fears of returning with diminished abilities. Survivors may return to their jobs but later be dismissed because they can no longer handle the responsibilities. After a brain injury, some people adjust well to the idea of not being able to work again and discover a sense of accomplishment and satisfaction in personal relationships, volunteering in the community, and other activities.

Those survivors able to return to work in the same job or in a new position may need retraining or job accommodations, such as more time to do tasks, a lighter work load, or specialized equipment. Some of them may also have difficulty with appropriate social skills, which can cause friction with co-workers or customers. Since a high level of fatigue is common among people with brain injury, they may be able to work only a few hours a day, at least in the beginning. (This kind of fatigue does not mean the survivor is not getting enough sleep. A healing brain grabs a great deal of energy from the body, so physical energy winds down quickly. In addition, the strain of handling cognitive tasks can be extreme, which leads to mental fatigue as well. Typically, fatigue becomes less of a problem over time.) This kind of situation requires that the survivor, employer, and co-workers understand what has happened (and even so, not everyone may be understanding or patient). Many elements are involved in returning to work after a brain injury. Doctors, therapists, and specialists such as job coaches and vocational rehabilitation counselors can assist you with this process.

```
The VA medical doctor says I am not work returnable. They ask
me questions and I answer. They sent me through MRI and EEG
testing. Have they told me why I am not work returnable? If so,
did their question appear to me to be a statement? Was their
statement a question? Was my answers so far off their questions
or what I thought was a question and with my chosen words and
slow speech that made no sense give them the reason to not be
able to allow me to return to work? Did I miss it all and they
see my blankness of confusion, lack of understanding? Do they not
know how to help me to get my brain to function fully again, so
```

are they writing me off? Is this why they said I am not work returnable? Am I so far out of touch with my injuries and lack of abilities that I have no ideas what they are? Why has no one told me? If someone did, why didn't I understand and know they were? I feel lost. If I was to return to work now, I don't know where or what I'd do. - **Todd**

☞ Here are some prompts for insight into yourself and your feelings about work:

Date: _____
- I have been told I will eventually be able to return to my job and…
- I have been told I will not be able to return to my job and…
- If I have to try another job…
- I have some limitations now that will affect my ability to work, and they are…
- I have some strengths that will help me when I return to work, and they are…
- Fatigue is a big problem for me right now, and…
- I returned to my job, but they let me go…
- I hope that if I cannot return to my old job but must find another one, I…
- I used to be the main breadwinner in my household, but that's no longer true. That makes me feel…
- Because my spouse has had to take over the role of main breadwinner, I…
- Because I cannot return to my old job, my family…
- My family could help me deal with the change in my job situation by…
- Having to go on disability because I can't return to work right now is…
- I'm afraid to return to work because…
- I'm excited to return to work because…
- Even if I am unable to return to work, I can still…
- Freewrite...

My Story 5-10
Back at Work

If you are able to return to work, either the same job or a new one, here are some prompts for you.

```
    Returning to my job after my injury was a hope for recovery
and fear of failure. I'm a software engineer so I must be able to
think in concepts. What I'm deeply grateful for is that my
company put me at the same desk, doing the same job, with the
same computer. My job was to work on regaining memory, not
learning new things. All things were new at that point. As I sat
at my desk and did things I found I had some recall of, it all
began to come back. Very slowly I found I did know how to do
things in a program and that brought my spirits up. I've never
gotten all the comfort with concepts back, at least not yet,
though it is easier now. Doing a procedure, one step at a time
kind of thing, is easy to learn and do. It doesn't take many
working memory cells for that and I do well. My work is more
limited but I'm still at it and others see me as adding value. It
makes me smile and glad I was able to continue working. - Phil
```

☞ Think about how your brain injury has affected your interest and ability to work.

Date:_____
- Returning to my job after my injury…
- Because I wasn't able to return to my old job but found a new one…
- Coming to a new place to work…
- I received the assistance I needed to work again and…
- People at work view me differently now because…
- I have discovered I can use my strengths on the job now, and they are…
- I have discovered some limitations at work that I didn't have before, and…
- I'm taking action to deal with my limitations on the job by…
- I feel I've had a successful day at work when…
- Today was a great day at work because…
- Work didn't go well today because…
- I'm going to work again, but I'm afraid because…
- To deal with my fears about going to my job, I…
- What I want my co-workers to understand about me is…
- What my boss needs to know about me is…
- What my boss and co-workers can do to help me is…
- At the end of my work day …
- Freewrite...

My Story 5-11
Back to School

A large number of brain injuries occur in young people still in high school and college. Other survivors who are older sometimes choose to return to school so they can follow a new career or vocational path. In either case, completing their education, if at all possible, can offer them a better future with more work choices. It is an important and worthwhile goal.

As with returning to work, it is important to have assistance from appropriate counselors and therapists, as well as school personnel, who can assist you with your return to the classroom.

☞ There are numerous variables involved in returning to school, only a few of which are covered here. Begin by writing about how they affect you.

Date: _____
- Returning to school after my brain injury…
- I've had difficulties in school since my brain injury because…
- My teachers and classmates…
- I don't want my teachers and classmates to know…
- Some things that have remained the same in school even after my brain injury are…
- Even though it will now take me longer to complete my education, I…
- I don't want to continue in school because…
- People at school view me differently now because…
- Some of the people who are helping me at school…
- It's so frustrating in school now because…
- I've noticed that my abilities in school…
- I'll stay in school until I'm done, no matter what, because…
- Freewrite...

My Story 5-12
Social Activities

Before your injury you were involved in various social activities, and depending on your level of recovery, you're probably looking forward to resuming this part of your life. However, you might face some new difficulties. Physical challenges might mean you can no longer join in activities such as bowling with your co-workers, going out dancing, running marathons—or even going to the movies. Those same challenges might make it harder for you merely to venture out of the house or get around town. Perhaps your friends have stopped calling or visiting, and you're not sure why. If you're not able to work, that cuts back on your ability to make new social contacts and makes it harder to stay in touch with old friends there. Perhaps fatigue, memory and cognitive problems, and a new inability to feel comfortable in social situations are also playing an unwelcome role. As with other areas of your life, please feel free to discuss this with a counselor or therapist or trusted family members and friends.

☞ Here are some prompts about social activities.

Date: _____

- In your journal, make a list with the title: "Activities I enjoyed before my injury." Then write as many as you can.

- Of those activities, I will again be able to…
- I'm hoping that I can once again ___(name activity)___, but…
- Before my injury, I used to ___(name activity)___, and I know I will do it again because…
- Before my injury, I used to ___(name activity)___, and I'm afraid I won't be able do it again because…
- My friends don't invite me along any more…
- Even if I can't resume all my old activities, I can still…
- As soon as I can ___(name activity)___, then I can also…
- It's difficult now for me to join in social activities because…
- Joining in social activities now…
- I can make new friends …
- A new activity I would like to try now is…
- Freewrite...

My Story 5-13
Giving of Yourself

If you're not yet able to return to work or school, you might be able to volunteer for an organization in your community. Being a volunteer offers many benefits. It can provide experience that might be useful when you return to work. It can allow you to use your abilities in a positive way and explore new skills. You will get out of the house and interact with a variety of people. Volunteering can help you feel more connected to the larger world and expand your horizons. And, last but not least, you can make a significant contribution to your community, perhaps in ways you had never before considered. When you volunteer, you help others—and you also help yourself.

```
   I have a second chance at life and I intend to live it out
with care, love and giving back to show that even though I was in
a terrible accident that I'm able to get up and be the best
father, son and citizen that I can be. I have used the spare time
that I have now to volunteer with the Humane Society, The VA
Hospital, and Habitat for Humanity. My sister-in-law is a Middle
School Special Education Teacher I come to realize that with my
special circumstances of being a Traumatic Brain Injury survivor,
I have real insight into the lives and challenge these beautiful
and special kids face on a daily basis. So I volunteer at the
school helping the kids with Special Olympics and doing things
like working with them on special life skills like cooking lunch.
   With my situation and where I've landed at I can really relate
to the kids and the special needs they face every day. And with
my 3 kids it gives me a chance to show my kids all the things
that I've taught and preached to them about if you fall down you
get up dust yourself off and keep moving in a forward direction,
with a positive attitude. - Michael
```

☞ Here are some prompts about volunteering:

Date: _____
- In your journal, make a list titled "Some places I might like to volunteer." Write as many as you can.

- I have so much to offer as a volunteer because…
- What I can offer as a volunteer is…
- I would like to volunteer because…
- Some tasks I would like to do as a volunteer are..
- I will investigate how I can become a volunteer by…
- The goals I have for being a volunteer are…
- Freewrite...

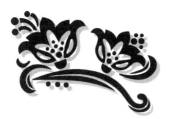

Chapter 6
Later On: Any Positives?

"It is then that you will hear a voice within yourself. It is there all the time, but you never listened before…it will grow louder and clearer the more you take heed of its message until one day it thunders inside you and you will have come home."
Kristin Zambucka, Ano, Ano

"We all suffered in our past. We all became wiser for it. In writing about past suffering, we can put that acquired wisdom to work, along with the story of how we emerged from it."
Robert Yehling, The Write Time

You have sustained a brain injury of some type. You are moving forward with your life and creating a new story for yourself. You have recovered well enough to journal with this workbook (or the original injury wasn't severe enough to prevent you from using it). In addition, you may now be able to live independently or you may need assistance of some type. Your life may be very similar to your life before the injury, or it may be extremely different. *You* may be very different. But whatever your situation, you survived a brain injury—you are alive. You are a valuable person entitled to a fulfilling life.

```
I am a brain injury survivor. - Todd
```

If you are working through your grief and making emotional adjustments to the changes you've experienced, you're likely feeling more realistic about your situation and hopeful about the future. You are coming to terms with what the injury means for you. At times—even frequently—you can enjoy the pleasure and beauty in your life. You're having some feeling of better control over events, along with greater self-confidence. You have the opportunity to make choices and are setting personal goals and pursuing them. You know you can't go back, and you know you must do the best you can with whatever abilities and skills you have now. Yes, you face challenges that can sometimes get the best of you (keep journaling!), but in this section of the workbook, you'll explore positive aspects of your post-injury life.

```
    Having such a severe accident made me realize how quickly a
    little thing like horses spooking can occur and how the life
    force can be snuffed as easily as we blow out a candle. Instead
    of waiting for life to begin, I changed the way I live. Every day
    is precious, like the first time I took a walk after I finally
    could. I went along familiar trails. It was after a good rain.
    All the plants sparkled as the sun lit up the drops clinging to
```

After Brain Injury: Telling Your Story 85

```
the leaves, twinkling like so many diamonds. I went to each plant
in amazement of the flowers, the leaves dancing in the breezes,
the trickle of water in the washes, the birds and rabbits and
lizards I saw. - Lesley
```

Remember that people with brain injury, like people in general, who see life as a glass half-full tend to do better than those who see it as half-empty. Those who do their best to remain positive and optimistic are likely to have better outcomes than those who sabotage themselves with anxiety and negativity. If you need help keeping your spirits up, create your own cheerleading squad—recruit your spouse or partner, parents, brothers or sisters, or good friends to encourage and support you. Let them know you want and need to deal with negative issues when necessary but to keep the overall focus on the positive. If necessary, work with a good counselor or therapist experienced in brain injury. Attend a support group for people with brain injuries to meet others who share your optimistic attitude and fighting spirit.

Positive thinking cannot change the fact that you have a brain injury. However, it can shape your attitudes and reactions to situations affected by the injury. For instance, if you refuse to work on the cognitive exercises your outpatient speech therapist gives you to do at home in between appointments, you may prevent yourself from recovering as well as you could have. On the other hand, say your occupational therapist knows you are able to start taking public transportation, and even though you are afraid at first, you face your fear and learn how to ride the bus. By keeping a positive attitude, you win more independence and assist your recovery.

Even small bits of positive attitude can help. If you frequently declare that you are becoming stronger, learning more coping skills, or adjusting to your new situation, those things will be more likely to happen than if you complain about feeling bad or focus on activities you can no longer do. Over time these small, positive affirmations build on one another to enhance your life.

Following are some journaling exercises to help you look on the brighter side. If you're not ready to write from these prompts yet, that's fine. Read through them and let their messages sink in so they can gently begin to work their magic. Or if you decide to use them but don't quite believe you can be positive enough, that's okay, too. Keep writing anyway, in whatever emotional state you find yourself. Date your entries and follow your progress. Many people, including survivors of brain injury, have improved their lives by patiently and consciously envisioning their futures, which is like drawing a map to an unknown destination and then trusting it to lead you there.

My Story 6-1
Your "Sports Pages"

U.S. Supreme Court Justice Earl Warren once said, "I always turn to the sports pages first, which record people's accomplishments. The front page has nothing but man's failures."

That's an excellent way to begin the day—reading about accomplishments rather than failures. Which path would you rather follow when thinking about yourself? Do you turn to your "sports pages"—your accomplishments—first? Or do you keep your failures front and center? Your choice can make a huge difference in your outlook and your life.

```
Today, my sports pages say that many of the things I've always
done, I can still do. Even though I can't do things as fast or
perhaps as accurately, I can still do them. As I learn more about
who I am now, I've become more comfortable with me. This seems to
balance well with learning about how to do the things I enjoy
along with how I earn a living. My woodshop was early on a very
hard place to return to. That set of skills I'd formed had seemed
to abandon me. I was concerned about no longer being able to have
any of the joy I'd previously felt there. Slowly my skills began
to return as an automatic sequence of movements. The joy returned
with that feeling of accomplishment. Perhaps the rest of my life
will come back online in much the same way. - Ken

My biggest accomplishment is that I'm still alive. - Shellee
```

☞ Use this prompt often, and it will become a running list of your accomplishments, which you can review whenever you need a boost.

Date: _____
- ✎ I often think of my own "sports pages" first, that list of all my accomplishments, and especially the ones I've made since my brain injury. Today, my sports pages say…
- ✎ Freewrite…

My Story 6-2
Your Better Stories

A few years ago, an article in *Ode* magazine had this title: "What the world needs now are better stories."

How true that is! In the popular media, most of the time and space are devoted to stories about what's wrong in the world. They may be true, but they're certainly not the *best* stories, simply because the media don't pay much attention to what is uplifting or good.

Beneath the article title was this tidbit: "We think the world is in bad shape. But the reality is that every moment of every day, all over the world, people are solving problems. That's why we need to do what we can to spread the kind of stories that make the world a more beautiful place." And then came the real point of the article: "The better story is not an illusion; it is a choice, a calling." (*Ode* magazine, April 2006)

So it is with you.

Even with a brain injury, you can often choose the stories you let into your mind by choosing what you read or watch or listen to. You can often choose what you let into your mind by making a conscious decision about the words you allow to run around up there. *You can choose your stories—even the ones you tell yourself about yourself.*

More than likely, you don't realize you can do this. No one taught you how, or gave you permission. But you have the ability to choose many of your thoughts—the stories you tell yourself. Jill Bolte Taylor, Ph.D., is a neuroanatomist who had a massive stroke that for a time wiped out her left brain functions, including the chatter inside her head (something we all have). She wrote about her experience in her book, *My Stroke of Insight*, explaining that the first step to finding inner peace is "making that internal decision that internal verbal abuse is not acceptable behavior." In an interview, she explained further:

"We've got this incessant brain chatter, and very few of us actually pay attention to what it is saying. We let these little personalities inside our brain say whatever they want. For me, it's that little voice critical of myself or of others. That little, mean person in there—I don't see any healthy, worthwhile, productive role for her to play in my life as a healthy adult. I have silenced that little voice inside of me, and I believe we all should. We're just not trained as a society that we have the right or the ability to censor our own brain and to take some responsibility for our thoughts and what thoughts grow and what thoughts don't. I'm very excited we're at a time when people are actually willing to…realize that their thoughts are these tiny groups of cells, which are the products of neurons, and that we have some say in which circuits run and which ones don't." *(Science of Mind*, Oct. 2008, interview by Barbara Stahura)

Take a few minutes sometime and listen to your thoughts, your self-talk. As with most people, it's likely that a large portion of your thoughts follow a habitual pattern day after day. And if you're like a number of people, many of those thoughts fall to the negative side. Is that true for you? Do you dwell on those things you can no longer do, or can't do as well, since your brain injury?

Are you forgetting to tell yourself the *best* stories about you? Stories about how you survived a brain injury and are working hard on your recovery. Stories about how you are a gift to the world, about how you have value and worth and unique perspectives. You are a miracle and will never know how much you contribute to the lives of others. Because you *do* contribute—even now. Remember that always.

You can choose to fall into the negative, or you can choose to tell your best story. You can change your self-talk and change your mind. Not every change of mind is dramatic, nor does it have to be. The changes can be tiny and still make a huge difference.

```
    A stampede of horses changed the story of my life by causing
me to focus on what is right here, right now. The brain injury I
experienced was severe enough to keep me hospitalized for 3 and
one half months then under nursing care at home for another
month….I appreciate more now and that lesson doesn't go away. I
cherish what I have and focus on the benefits of the friends and
family around me. My brain injury was a life affirming experience
for me. - Lesley

    One of my best stories about myself is that I know that my
past difficulties have made me a stronger person because I am
still kick'n.  Several of my friends pointed out when I lived
through falling 6 meters onto my head… "you cannot deny being
hard headed anymore!"  What are friends there for if not to point
out your flaws?  Am I hard headed or am I intentional?  I AM a
survivor of a lot of things.  AND  I am a thriver! I live in
paradise!  I did not plan that either! - Lela
```

☞ Use these prompts often to reinforce the positives and accomplishments in your life:

Date: _____
- One of my best stories about myself is…
- I used to have mostly negative stories about myself, but I made them more positive by…
- Even though I can no longer do some of the things I used to, I can still…
- It's harder for me now to do some things, but I still…
- I treat myself with kindness and patience by…
- One tiny thing I did to change my self-talk from negative to positive was…
- One huge thing I did to change my self-talk from negative to positive was…
- Something I now refuse to believe about myself is…
- Some steps I can take to change my negative self-talk to positive self-talk is…
- Freewrite...

My Story 6-3
Time Capsule Treasures, Part 1

Everyone has treasures they cherish, which could be material objects, loved ones, special places, pieces of music, books, and even intangible items such as religious faith or certain memories. What are some of the treasures you cherish? If you were asked to put some of them in a time capsule that only you could open in five years, which ones would you choose? What would they say about you and how you were handling your new, post-injury life?

```
    I was asked to put a few of my treasures in a time capsule
that only I will be able to open in five years. A treasure I
choose is the memory of having deep meaningful talks while
sitting in warm sudsy water and seeing the Catalinas
[mountains]out the windows from the tub in our master bath. These
are times worth remembering because they are part of letting
another see beneath the shell each of us can hold as the face we
wear. Long ago I didn't realize I held a mask. I thought I was
the mask. Knowing better than that lets me shine as myself and no
longer as someone else. - Ken
```

Writing about your treasures can help you feel happier and encourage you to stay positive. If the treasures cannot literally be put in a time capsule—such as the cabin in the mountains where you spent summers with your grandparents or the memory of your late husband—imagine that you can put absolutely anything in there. After all, this is your journal, and you can imagine whatever you want in its pages!

☞ You can use all three of these prompts one after the other, or you can write from the first one and then come back to the others after some time has passed. For each one, you can make a list or write in full sentences.

Date: _____
☞ Part 1
✎ I was asked to put a few of my treasures in a time capsule that only I will be able to open in five years. The treasures I choose are…

Date: _____
☞ Part 2 Now imagine yourself five years in the future:
✎ Five years have passed, and I open the time capsule with my treasures in it. As I take them out, I…

Date: _____
☞ Part 3 At some other time in the future:
✎ I'm going to add new or different items to my time capsule treasures. This time around, I choose…

My Story 6-4
Time Capsule Treasures, Part 2

There are other ways to do this exercise. Get out your markers, crayons, or colored pencils. In your journal, draw a time capsule that you can fill with drawings of your treasures. See example below. You can draw circles inside the capsule and fill them with words to describe the treasures. You can even cut pictures from magazines to paste into your journal as a collage.

Be sure to put a label on the time capsule with "Today's date" and "Five years from today's date." That will project your imagination forward in time so you can anticipate the future in a positive way.

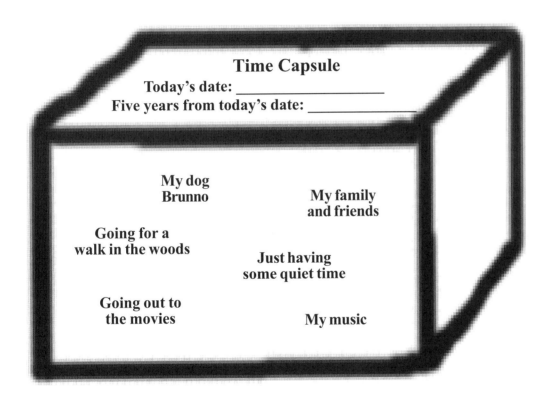

My Story 6-5
No One Can Take This Away From Me

Everyone has qualities, beliefs, or elements of their lives that will remain with them always, no matter what. Perhaps it's religious faith, or an unshakable belief in one's self to persevere. Maybe it's a parent's or a child's love, or maintaining a sense of humor even in the face of dire circumstances.

```
   I know I'm still here because God has something for me to do.
```
- **Michael**

☞ What is something that no one can take away from you? Even now, after a brain injury, what quality, belief, or other element of your life remains as strong as ever? Or perhaps you have developed a new quality that is sending out tender roots inside you, and you want to nurture and protect it as it grows strong. How would you do that?

Date: _____

🖋 One thing that no one will ever be able to take away from me is…
🖋 I have total faith in…
🖋 Something or someone that continues to support me now is…
🖋 Since my injury, I have developed a new strength, quality, or some element of my life that can keep me strong, and it…
🖋 Freewrite...

My Story 6-6
Invitation

On some days you may feel as if your strengths or positive beliefs have taken a hike and left you at home. You feel lost without them and can't find them anywhere. It's possible they needed to rest for a while, or maybe they're hibernating until conditions improve, like bears waiting out the harsh winter by sleeping until spring brings a gentler season. If this is the case, issue an invitation to entice them back out into the open where you can depend upon them once again.

```
    I want to invite working memory into my life now because
sometimes it's difficult to talk to people when I have trouble
remembering what I say. I use the wrong words or no word come out
just noises. When I talk with people that rush me to find my
words or won't tell me what the topic was again that's negative
and frustrating. I like talking with my son. If I muse [mess] up
my words or forget what we were talking about, he joking tells
me, points it out, and reminds me. And we juckel [chuckle] &
laugh about it. Sometimes about from my muse up from days before.
That's positive and light no pressure. It helps my memory get
better and lets me know what I need to work on to get it better.
Thank you son I love you. - Todd
```

☞ Use this prompt as many times as necessary for as many qualities or strengths, people or activities you wish to invite:

Date: _____
🖉 I want to invite _____ into my life right now because...
🖉 Freewrite...

My Story 6-7
RSVP

After you send out your invitations, imagine what kind of responses you'll get. Do your invitees (human or otherwise) agree to come back with pleasure? Or do they dig in their heels and refuse to return? Perhaps some would like to re-enter your life but aren't quite sure if it's the right time, so they need a bit of encouragement.

If you want to know more about their responses, one way to clarify matters is to write a dialogue. You've already used this format (see "Talking with Your Brain," My Story 1-5, Chapter 1 for a reminder). Remember that both sides of the dialogue come from your own imagination—a technique that can reveal quite a lot about yourself and your situation.

- ☞ It's helpful to do your relaxation technique. During that time, silently ask your dialogue "partner" what it might want to reveal during the writing and thank it for being honest with you.

→ Begin with relaxation technique. Refer to page 10.

Date: _____
- ☞ Insert quality, person, etc. you are dialoging with:
- ✎ Me:
  (Dialogue Partner's Name:)

- ✎ Freewrite...

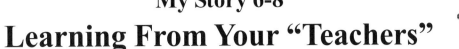

My Story 6-8
Learning From Your "Teachers"

Part of being human is being able to use what you have learned from the past in order to move more confidently into the future. "Teachers" are all around you. They can be your progress and successes, as well as mistakes and missteps. You can learn from other people, nature, books and movies, and events and situations. Even your thoughts—those stories you tell yourself—can be your teachers once you're able to tune into what they're saying. Over time and through trial and error, you will discover what works and what doesn't, what brings satisfaction or drives you crazy with frustration. This ability to learn from experiences can be hampered, sometimes greatly, by a brain injury, but since you are using this workbook you likely still retain it to some degree. If you can learn to spot your "teachers" and use the resources they offer, you can continue to make progress in your own ways.

```
My teachers are
1. my dog Petey
2. my mom and dad
3. favorite TV show, Bones
4. Dr. Thomas, my neurologist
5. the nurses at the clinic
6. Becca, my best friend who sticks by me
7. the baby robins in the tree outside my bedroom window
8. library books
9. walking outside
10. speech therapy
```
- **Hannah**

```
Walking outside is teaching me again that the world is a
beautiful place, even in my own city. I can see how the seasons
change one after the other, and they never miss when it's their
turn to come around again. They are faithful. They stick by each
other, like Becca sticks by me. Even though my other friends
don't call anymore since my accident. When I walk outside I have
to go slow but nature doesn't mind. It's there all around me and
has no place to go so it's patient. I'm trying to be patient with
myself.
```
- **Hannah**

Remember that progress after a brain injury can come in baby steps, even micro-steps, as well as in occasional leaps. You might not advance at an even pace. Your progress might occur in a stairstep fashion where you make a big jump, then plateau for a time, followed by another jump. Everyone's healing and recovery is different, so let yours teach you.

☞ Here are some prompts about learning from your "teachers." Once you start searching your world for teachers, you will find more and more. There is always something more to learn!

Date: _____

✎ In your journal, write the numbers from 1-10 and make a list of your "teachers."

☞ Now, using this list of teachers, you can write about them individually or write about them as a group. The more teachers you find, the more you'll return to this exercise.

✎ __(Name of teacher)__ is teaching me…
✎ __(Name of teacher)__ has already taught me…

☞ Do you want to keep learning from these teachers, or not? Why?
(Use this prompt for as many teachers as you like.)

✎ I want to keep learning from __(Name of teacher)__ because…
✎ I prefer not to learn anymore from __(Name of teacher)__ because…
✎ Freewrite...

My Story 6-9
Being a Teacher

You can be a teacher, too. In fact, you probably already are and don't know it. People often teach by example, even when they don't realize that others are paying attention. You are a teacher for your children, for instance, as they watch how you handle situations in daily life. You might also be an example for adults. Say you attend rehab therapy sessions, and your therapist takes you to the mall so you can practice navigating through crowds and making the right purchases. You might unintentionally teach other shoppers the value of determination and persistence in the face of adversity.

Of course, you can teach on purpose as well. It's not necessary to go on the public speaking circuit or make a big deal out of this—excellent teaching is often quiet and unassuming. What have you learned from living with your brain injury that you could share with your family and friends, other survivors, or even strangers you meet out in the world? What do you want them to know about your brain injury and how it changed your life? What would you like them to know about how you are still the same person? In addition, teaching does not always require words: How do you act when faced with difficulty or a challenge?

☞ Use the prompts to write about how you can become a teacher:

Date: _____
- Some things I could teach or tell others about are…
- I could do this by…
- In my heart, I know the most important thing I want to teach others about is…
- Freewrite…

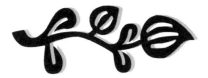

Chapter 7
Miscellaneous Prompts

*"To name the world in your own terms, to tell your own story,
is an act of authority and power. When you write, you are saying, in effect,
'I have a voice. I have a story. This is what I have to say.'"*
Rebecca McClanahan, *Write Your Heart Out*

"… life is a universe of fragments yearning for coherence."
Kim Stafford, *The Muses Among Us*

This last section of the workbook is a collection of miscellaneous prompts for you to use any time you feel like expressing yourself through writing. Each one of them will help you use your voice and tell your story. Your writing with these prompts could reveal significant insights or small tidbits of information, or it might simply be relaxing. It's all valuable.

It is likely that your responses to some of the more open-ended prompts will change every time you go back to them, such as "I will…" or "I would love to..." Your responses to some of the more directed prompts could remain the same, or nearly so, as with "Something I've never told anyone is…" Remember, whatever you write at any given time is fine.

As with the other prompts in this workbook, you can return to these as often as you like. It's enlightening to look back at your past journal entries, to see how you have changed and to track the progress you have made—or to see where you are stuck and might need a boost to get out of a rut.

These prompts don't require any explanation, and they are listed one after the other. Be sure to date each entry in your journal in order to track your thoughts over time. If you choose, set your timer and as much as possible keep your pen moving for the entire time. This technique allows more insights and information to rise to the surface, which can reveal some helpful surprises.

When you see three dots (…) inside a prompt, it means you should fill in the blank and then continue writing from the prompt. Here's an example: For "I feel good about…because…" someone might write, "I feel good about eating ice cream because…"

When you use this section, you can choose a prompt that appeals to you at that moment. Or you can challenge yourself by flipping through the pages, closing your eyes and pointing to a prompt at random. Remember that you can use the techniques you used in the earlier sections of the workbook, such as creating lists, writing a dialogue, or "Using the Senses to Remember," My Story 2-13, Chapter 2.

☞ Use whatever technique appeals to you, and feel free to make up your own.

- I will…
- I won't…
- I feel…
- I believe…
- I can't…

- I can…
- I would love to…
- I never want to…
- I'm most worried about…
- If I could free my mind…
- The qualities I most appreciate in myself are … because…
- A bad habit I'd like to eliminate is … because…
- If I could make a movie of my life, it would…
- Tomorrow when I step outsde my door, I…
- Why should I have to…
- The place where I find the most peace is … because… (This is an excellent prompt to use with "Using the Senses to Remember," My Story 2-13, Chapter 2)
- A place that I'd rather not return to is … because…
- My hero today is … because
- A childhood hero of mine was … because…
- I am a hero to … because…
- Hanging in my closet are…
- In my kitchen cabinets are...
- I promise myself I will…
- I want…
- I know…
- Something I've never told anyone is…
- I want the whole world to know…
- I strive to do my best when…
- I don't care if I ever do my best for…
- Something I accomplished today was…
- I like…
- I hate…
- I love…
- I was so nervous when…
- I felt so strong when…
- When I was young I wanted to…
- My life would have been different if I…
- Today I…
- I ask (name) to forgive me for…
- I forgive (name) for…
- My goal for today is…
- My goal for next month is…
- My goal for the next year is…
- I could never repay (person) because…
- A story about a "lump of coal" in my life that turned into a "diamond" is…
- I feel good about … because…
- I always feel sad when…
- Some days my life feels like I'm forced to dig a long ditch in the hot sun because…
- Some days my life feels like a holiday because…
- One self-defeating thought I have often is…
- One thought that always lifts me up is…
- I remember what it was like to…
- An act of kindness I'll remember for a long time is…

- I don't understand how someone could be so mean as to…
- When things don't go my way, I…
- When someone else is having a bad day, I…
- When (name) hurt my feelings, I…
- When I hurt (name's) feelings, I…
- If I knew I could not fail, I would…
- Something that fear of failure keeps me from doing is…
- A mistake I never want to make again is…
- When I go to the grocery store, I can't seem to stay away from … because…
- When I go to the mall, I can't seem to stay away from … because…
- If I won the lottery, I would…
- If I had only $5 to my name, I would…
- I believe in miracles because…
- There is no such thing as miracles because…
- Today is…
- Yesterday was…
- These days a hard day's work for me is…
- In the past, a hard day's work for me was…
- Something in myself I would like to improve is…
- Something in myself I'm satisfied with is…
- I have never thanked (person) for … because…
- When (person) lost his/her temper with me, I…
- When I lost my temper with (person), I…
- Something I can do to control my temper better is…
- I like losing my temper because…
- When I am alone and quiet, I can't help thinking about…
- It's okay to keep thinking about … because…
- It's not okay to keep thinking about … because…
- Something I will always love about myself is…
- Something I will always love about (person or thing) is…
- When I was young, my parents told me to never … but I did it anyway, and…
- When I was young, my parents told me to never … and I never did it because…
- Some of the thoughts I think over and over again are…
- My family drives me crazy because…
- My family takes good care of me because…
- I can learn and grow from bad times if I…
- It's better to learn and grow from good times because…
- My life is a journey to…
- The last time I laughed at myself…
- When people push me too hard, I…
- The people who have remained my friends…
- At the last social gathering I attended, I…
- If I can't have … I can be happy instead with … because…
- Today, one thing I want from life is…
- Today, one thing I never want to have in my life again is…
- I welcome … into my life because…
- Today I am grateful for…
- In the future I will be grateful for…
- I have recovered from…

- ✎ A dream I wish I had is…
- ✎ A dream I wish I had never had is…
- ✎ I no longer believe in…
- ✎ I will always believe in…

☞ We have included a few lined pages for you to begin your journaling. See page 107.

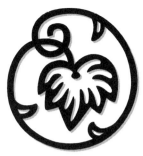

Chapter 8
Journaling in a Group

Journaling is usually a private activity, so that the journaler feels totally free to write about anything. Generally, journalers do not share their writings with others. Yet sometimes people come together to journal in a group in order to find support and kinship. They often discover a special kind of shared energy there that does not appear when journaling alone. This workbook began as a journaling group for people with brain injury, to see if they would find any benefit in writing about and sharing their experiences with one another. Most, if not all, of our participants had a positive experience and asked to return again. They enjoyed being able to explore their lives after brain injury in a friendly, non-clinical setting with a creative technique they had not tried before. They also found companionship with other people with brain injury, who could understand them better than anyone else.

People with brain injury can join together on their own in a journaling group, or therapists and trained journaling facilitators can help to create and lead a group. Here are some guidelines we found important for our journaling groups.

Respect

Respect for others in the group and their writing is crucial. Journaling can reveal private and difficult subjects, so it is essential that no one in the group or their writing be judged in a negative way by anyone else.

Confidentiality

Confidentiality is important. Group participants should agree to not reveal anything said or done within the journaling group to anyone outside the group. If necessary, a brief reminder at the start of every session can help reinforce this.

Note: Confidentiality of group sessions is important. However, if a participant makes a threat to another person or indicates intentions to harm himself, then concern for the safety of all participants overrides confidentiality. In this situation, the group leaders are responsible for reporting their concerns to family and/or professionals to protect the well-being of the individuals involved.

Reading aloud

In journaling groups, participants often read their writing aloud to the group. Remember, however, that this is absolutely voluntary. Those who do not want to share their writing should not be pressured to do so in any way.

Discussion

It's likely that some discussion will happen after a round of reading aloud. This is an excellent way for participants to connect with each other. Just be prepared to gently keep people on track if they veer off too far. It's common that at least one person in the group will want to talk a lot more than anyone else, so also be ready to kindly interrupt and move the group on.

Tools

Everyone should have the appropriate tools for journaling—a copy of this book, a notebook or journal to write in, pens or pencils (or laptop computer), and sometimes crayons or colored pencils or markers (boxes of these can be shared).

Relaxation Exercise

It's helpful to do a short relaxation exercise or meditation at the beginning of each group meeting (see page 10 for an example or use your own). About 5 minutes is a good length of time, but feel free to do what works for the group. Relaxing like this allows everyone to become more fully present and to shake off the cares of the day. If you have a music player handy, you can play soft instrumental music during the relaxation time.

Time Sessions

Be sure to time the writing sessions, ranging up to 20 minutes, depending on the available time and the abilities of people in the group. (In our groups, the usual writing time was 15-20 minutes. Some participants could fill up an entire page in that time, while others wrote only a few sentences.) It can be helpful to announce when there is a minute left to go in the session so people can wrap up their thoughts. In our 90-minute meetings, we were able to do two or three writing sessions, with reading and a little discussion in between each one.

Explain Prompts

If someone in the group does not understand the prompt being used, explain it in more detail or perhaps suggest another topic that works better for that person.

Be Flexible

If someone prefers to write about something other than the prompt at hand, that's perfectly fine. People should be allowed to write about whatever is on their minds.

Brain Injury Resources

Books and CDs
These are only a few of the many resources available about the human brain and brain injury. You can check with your local library or bookstore and search Amazon.com to find them and many others. You can also contact local and state Brain Injury Associations and rehabilitation hospitals in your area.

Living with Brain Injury
Stephen Gurgevich, Ph.D., *Brain Injury Healing*; a CD that demonstrates the use of self-hypnosis for tapping into the mind-body connection to promote more rapid healing after a brain injury. To order, call 866-506-1700.

Douglas J. Mason and Jean-Louis Gottfried, *The Mild Traumatic Brain Injury Workbook: Your Program for Regaining Cognitive Function & Overcoming Emotional Pain*; New Harbinger Publications (2004)

Richard Senelick, M.D., and Karla Dougherty, *Living with Brain Injury: A Guide for Families*; Delmar Cengage Learning (2001)

Memoirs by and about survivors of brain injury
Janelle Breese Biagioni, *A Change of Mind: One Family's Journey through Brain Injury*; Lash and Associates Publishing/Training (2004)

Cathy Crimmins, *Where is the Mango Princess?*; Vintage (2001)

Ruthann Knechel Johansen, *Listening in the Silence, Seeing in the Dark: Reconstructing Life After Brain Injury*; University of California Press (2002)

PJ Long, *Gifts from the Broken Jar: Rediscovering Hope, Beauty, and Joy*; Equilibrium Press (2004)

Michael Paul Mason, *Head Cases: Stories of Brain Injury and its Aftermath*; Farrar, Straus and Giroux (2009)

Claudia L. Osborn, *Over My Head: A Doctor's Own Story Of Head Injury From the Inside Looking Out*; Andrews McMeel Publishing (2000)

Carolyn Rocchio, *Ketchup on the Baseboard: Rebuilding Life After Brain Injury*; Lash and Associates Publishing/Training (2004)

Madonna Siles, *Brain, Heal Thyself: A Caregiver's New Approach to Recovery from Stroke, Aneurysm, and Traumatic Brain Injuries*; Hampton Roads Publishing Company, Inc. (2006)

Floyd Skloot, *In the Shadow of Memory;* Bison Books (2004)

Barbara Stahura, *What I Thought I Knew*; Wyatt-MacKenzie Publishing, Inc. (2008)

Kara L. Swenson, *I'll Carry the Fork! Recovering a Life After Brain Injury;* Rising Star Press (1999)

Jill Bolte Taylor, Ph.D., *My Stroke of Insight*; Plume (2009)

Lee and Bob Woodruff, *In an Instant: A Family's Journey of Love and Healing*; Random House Trade Paperbacks (2008)

Journaling and Personal Storytelling

Kathleen Adams, *Journal to the Self: Twenty-Two Paths to Personal Growth - Open the Door to Self-Understanding by Writing, Reading, and Creating a Journal of Your Life*; Grand Central Publishing (1990)

Christina Baldwin, *Storycatcher: Making Sense of Our Lives Through the Power and Practice of Story*; New World Library (2007)

Christina Baldwin, *Life's Companion: Journal Writing as a Spiritual Quest*; Bantam (1990)

John Fox, CPT, *Finding What You Didn't Lose: Expressing Your Truth and Creativity Through Poem-Making*; Tarcher (1995)

Natalie Goldberg, *Writing Down the Bones: Freeing the Writer Within*; Shambhala (2005)

James Pennebaker, Ph.D., *Opening Up: The Healing Power of Expressing Emotions*; The Guilford Press (1997)

Date: _____

Date: _____

Date: _____

Date: _____

Date: _____

Date: _____